OXFORD HANDBOOKS IN EME[
Series Editors   R. N. Illingworth, C. E. Ro[

OXFORD HANDBOOKS IN EMERGENCY MEDICINE

This series has already established itself as the essential reference series for staff in A & E departments.

Each book begins with an introduction to the topic, including epidemiology where appropriate. The clinical presentation and the immediate practical management of common conditions are described in detail, enabling the casualty officer or nurse to deal with the problem on the spot. Where appropriate a specific course of action is recommended for each situation and alternatives discussed. Information is clearly laid out and easy to find— important for situations where swift action may be vital.

Details on when, how, and to whom to refer patients are covered, as well as the information required at referral, and what this information is used for. The management of the patient after referral to a specialist is also outlined.

The text of each book is supplemented with checklists, key points, clear diagrams illustrating practical procedures, and recommendations for further reading.

The Oxford Handbooks in Emergency Medicine are an invaluable resource for every member of the A & E team, written and edited by clinicians at the sharp end.

Anaesthesia and Analgesia in Emergency Medicine, Second Edition

Karen A. Illingworth F.R.C.A.
Accident and Emergency Department,
St James's University Hospital, Leeds

and

Karen H. Simpson F.R.C.A.
Department of Anaesthesia,
St James's University Hospital, Leeds

Illustrations by

Sue Swales
Accident and Emergency Department,
St James's University Hospital, Leeds

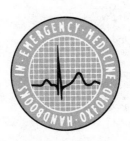

Oxford • New York • Tokyo
OXFORD UNIVERSITY PRESS
1998

2/98

37663528

Oxford University Press, Great Clarendon Street, Oxford OX2 6DP

Oxford   New York
Toronto
Athens   Auckland   Bangkok   Bogota   Bombay
Buenos Aires   Calcutta   Cape Town   Dar es Salaam
Delhi   Florence   Hong Kong   Istanbul   Karachi
Kuala Lumpur   Madras   Madrid   Melbourne
Mexico City   Nairobi   Paris   Singapore
Taipei   Tokyo   Toronto   Warsaw
and associated companies in
Berlin   Ibadan

Oxford is a trade mark of Oxford University Press

Published in the United States
by Oxford University Press Inc., New York

First edition published 1994

A catalogue record for this book is available from the British Library

Library of Congress Cataloging in Publication Data
Illingworth, Karen A.
Anaesthesia and analgesia in emergency medicine/Karen A.
Illingworth and Karen H. Simpson; illustrations by Sue Swales.–2nd ed.
(Oxford handbooks in emergency medicine; 18)
Includes bibliographical references and index.
1. Anaesthesia–Handbooks, manuals, etc.   2. Analgesia–Handbooks,
manuals, etc.   3. Emergency medicine–Handbooks, manuals, etc.
I. Simpson, Karen H.   II. Title.   III. Series.
[DNLM: 1. Emergencies–handbooks.   2. Anaesthesia–handbooks.
3. Analgesia–handbooks.   WB 39 098 v. 18 1998]
RD82.2.I43 1998   617.9'6042–dc21   97–41376
ISBN 0 19 262909 3 (Hbk)
ISBN 0 19 262908 5 (Pbk)

Typeset by Footnote Graphics, Warminster, Wiltshire

Printed in Great Britain by Bookcraft (Bath) Ltd, Midsomer Norton, Avon

Preface

This book concerns the provision of anaesthesia and analgesia for patients presenting as emergencies. Patients commonly come to the Accident and Emergency (A & E) department with pain problems or with conditions requiring local or general anaesthesia. Close cooperation between the staff of the anaesthesia and A & E departments is required if anaesthesia and analgesia are to be dealt with efficiently and safely. This book provides a concise guide to anaesthesia and pain relief in emergency medicine. The emphasis is on practical management of problems and clear instructions about the treatment of common conditions. This book is aimed at those working in multidisciplinary traumatology.

We are grateful to Dr Robin Illingworth for his invaluable advice and assistance in the preparation of this book. Thanks are also due to Sue Swales for skilfully turning our ideas into illustrations.

Leeds   K.A.I.
October 1997   K.H.S.

Contents

Part 1
General concepts of anaesthesia and analgesia

Part 1
General concepts of anaesthesia and analgesia

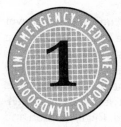

CHAPTER 1

General anaesthesia in the A & E department

Key points in general anaesthesia in the A & E department

- Problems can occur with any anaesthetic technique. There is no such thing as a 'simple' anaesthetic.
- All injured patients are at risk of regurgitation and aspiration of gastric contents during anaesthesia or recovery.
- Thorough preoperative history and examination may prevent anaesthetic problems.
- Preoperative resuscitation is mandatory.
- The anaesthetist must plan the anaesthetic technique after consultation about the proposed surgery. Adequate facilities must be available, including trained assistance for the anaesthetist.
- Guidelines must be available for the management of anaesthetic emergencies.
- A & E staff should be aware of and trained to assist with common anaesthetic emergencies.

Introduction

There is a danger of assuming that general anaesthesia in the A & E department for quick, simple procedures, will also be quick, simple, and thus suitable for very junior anaesthetists. Nothing could be further from the truth. When considering general anaesthesia neither 'simple' nor 'quick' should ever be thought synonymous with 'safe'. The simplest, quickest anaesthetic can still go wrong, with catastrophic results.

There are many problems associated with emergency general anaesthesia in the A & E department. Delayed gastric emptying commonly occurs with trauma, and may be potentiated by the use of opioids preoperatively. Regurgitation and aspiration of gastric contents may occur during anaesthesia or recovery. The need for fluid replacement may have been underestimated. Additional injuries may only become apparent at a later stage. Patients are often unpremedicated, and may expect to be discharged from hospital a few hours postoperatively. Lateral or prone positions may be required. Surgery sometimes exceeds its estimated duration as a result of unexpected findings. An accurate medical history may be difficult to obtain, particularly in the elderly patient. There may be doubt about medication and compliance; doses are easily missed in the time following injury. Previously undiagnosed medical problems are sometimes discovered. Emergency anaesthesia is often performed during the evening or night, when senior help may not be so readily available. Emergency anaesthesia is full of pitfalls for the unsuspecting anaesthetist. The following questions must be addressed before embarking on emergency general anaesthesia:

1. What surgery is required and which surgeon will be performing it?

2. When is the best time for the patient to have the operation? This may not be the most convenient time for the surgeon or anaesthetist!

3. What is the best anaesthetic technique to use, bearing in mind the surgery required, the surgeon performing it, and the patient's age, underlying medical conditions, and associated injuries? What if the patient may not be admitted to hospital postoperatively? Would a local anaesthetic technique be better than general anaesthesia?

4. Are the facilities and staff in the A & E department adequate for what is required, or should the operation be performed in a main operating theatre?

5. Do I feel confident in undertaking the case, or should I be seeking senior advice first?

Standards of care defined for anaesthesia in an operating theatre must be applied in the A & E setting, where a consultant anaesthetist should take responsibility. Guidelines should be established for selecting patients suitable for anaesthesia in the A & E department, preparation of patients, checking and servicing of anaesthesia and monitoring equipment, and recovery of anaesthetized or sedated patients. Instructions for dealing with rare emergencies such as malignant hyperthermia should be readily available. These must include details on how to obtain emergency drugs. Assistance for the anaesthetist must be provided by trained Operating Department Practitioners. Patients recovering from anaesthesia must be supervized by properly trained staff.

The facilities for giving general anaesthesia or sedation in A & E departments vary from hospital to hospital, from a dedicated major theatre to a minor operations theatre. The emergency theatre in the A & E department must be easily accessible, and of sufficient size to accommodate a wide variety of procedures. There must be adequate equipment and suitably trained operating department personnel to assist the anaesthetist at all times. Two other people apart from the anaesthetist must be present during general anaesthesia, so that the patient can be rapidly turned into the lateral position if regurgitation occurs. The A & E department is often a very isolated area for an unsupervised junior anaesthetist. There should be clear instructions about how to summon senior anaesthetic help in case of difficulty arising during anaesthesia.

The A & E doctor can help the anaesthetist by a good history and examination. It is essential for the anaesthetist to have as much relevant information as possible. Associated injuries must be clearly documented; for example, the anaesthetist must know if a patient requiring anaesthesia for reduction of a Colles fracture has also sustained a head injury. All preoperative treatment must be clearly documented, since drugs given may affect the response to anaesthesia. It is helpful, if the surgeon is aware of potential anaesthetic problems and their management. The anaesthetist should be given adequate warning of the need to administer an anaesthetic in the A & E department, so that full preoperative assessment and checking of equipment can be carried out. Although anaesthesia for such cases may be perceived as a low priority in comparison to other 'emergencies', the anaesthetist must try to arrange a definite time to attend, and if necessary delegate this duty to a colleague. Undue delay is unpleasant and detrimental to the patient, who may have been starved for many hours. Delay is also disruptive to the running of the A & E department, and leads to a poor relationship between the departments. The key to success is good communication between the A & E and Anaesthetic departments, and a mutual appreciation of the difficulties experienced by each.

Anaesthesia for children

Special consideration should be given to anaesthesia for children in the A & E department. Their needs differ from those of adults. An empathic approach by staff is essential for good paediatric anaesthesia. It is important to avoid keeping children waiting for procedures, since waiting makes them more anxious and hungrier. The anaesthetist should meet the child with at least one parent so that the child can see the parent accepting the anaesthetist. Most of the attention should be directed at the child, taking care to make eye contact and establish trust. Special attention should be given to the silent child, who may be more traumatized by the experience than the more noisy child. It is important to talk to the child in simple terms in a way that the child can understand. Truthfully and simply explain what is going to happen. It is not helpful to present children with difficult choices such as 'mask or needle'. It is better not to uncover children until necessary as this makes them feel more insecure. Allowing children a toy to play with whilst inducing anaesthesia may help. It is now accepted practice to have a parent present during the induction of anaesthesia. However, if a parent is reluctant it is probably best not to force the issue. Parents need to know what will happen during induction of anaesthesia and that they will be asked to leave as soon as their child is asleep. Parents should be allowed to rejoin their child as soon after the procedure as is practical.

The anaesthetist and the A & E department

The anaesthetist can be involved in the work of the A & E department by taking part in:

(1) anaesthesia for minor procedures, such as drainage of abscesses, manipulation of fractures, or cardioversion;

(2) management of airway problems, such as facial trauma, epiglottitis, or thermal injury to the airway;

(3) management of respiratory failure;

(4) management of the unconscious patient;

(5) management of the poisoned patient;

(6) resuscitation of the seriously ill or traumatized patient;

(7) transfer of patients to the Intensive Care Unit or inter-hospital transfer of sick patients; and

(8) major incidents.

Principles of general anaesthesia

General anaesthesia involves the production of sleep, analgesia, and relaxation using a variety of drugs and techniques. In the early days of anaesthesia, nitrous oxide and volatile agents such as ether provided all three facets of anaesthesia. Guedel described the four stages and planes of anaesthesia, and the anaesthetist relied on physical signs to judge the onset and depth of anaesthesia.

1. The first stage (analgesia) occurs from the beginning of induction of anaesthesia to loss of consciousness.

2. The second stage (excitement) occurs from loss of consciousness to the start of automatic breathing. Struggling, breath-holding, and vomiting may occur during this phase, and it is important to try to minimize the time spent in this stage.

3. The third stage (surgical anaesthesia) occurs from the start of automatic breathing to respiratory paralysis, and is subdivided into four planes, which are defined by

physical signs such as increasing paralysis of muscles (eye, intercostal, and diaphragmatic) and loss of reflex responses.

4. The fourth stage of anaesthesia (over-dosage) occurs from the onset of diaphragmatic paralysis to apnoea and death.

Stages 1 to 3 are seen in reverse order during recovery from anaesthesia.

The advent of intravenous induction agents, strong opioids, and muscle relaxants led to the development of balanced anaesthesia, where different drugs are used to produce the triad of sleep, analgesia, and relaxation. Intravenous induction agents produce anaesthesia rapidly, and patients pass through stages 1 and 2 very quickly. The advantages of a reduction in the time spent in stage 2 are obvious; however, it must be remembered that protective reflexes are lost very quickly, and that aspiration of gastric contents is a risk. It is important that the principles of the four stages of anaesthesia are understood, and that anaesthetists are trained to judge the depth of anaesthesia from physical signs. No one should touch an anaesthetized patient until the anaesthetist indicates that surgical anaesthesia has been achieved, because stimulation during light anaesthesia (stage 2) may produce coughing, laryngospasm, and vomiting. The use of muscle relaxants allows positive pressure ventilation and surgery at much lighter planes of surgical anaesthesia than are possible when using a volatile agent alone. The anaesthetist relies on experience and physical signs such as lachrymation, sweating, and cardiovascular changes to judge the depth of anaesthesia. However, muscle relaxants and strong opioids remove some of the physical signs of light anaesthesia, and awareness is a risk. Small concentrations of a volatile anaesthetic agent are used during balanced anaesthesia to reduce this risk.

Morbidity and mortality from anaesthesia

Minor morbidity includes headache, sore throat, damage to mouth or teeth, vomiting, sedation, confusion, temporary neuropraxia, and muscle pains. Although these problems are classified as minor, many patients remember and fear them. They are often mentioned during preoperative assessment. Every effort should be made to reduce these complications. Intermediate morbidity includes prolonged vomiting, pulmonary embolus, myocardial infarction, and chest infection. These conditions prolong hospital stay, and some may have permanent implications for the patient. Large-scale studies are required to assess the contribution of anaesthesia to these conditions and evaluate preventive methods. Major morbidity includes hepatorenal failure and the chronic vegetative state which results from prolonged cerebral hypoxaemia.

The safety of anaesthesia is estimated by large scale studies of mortality after surgery or maternal deaths. In 1949 the Association of Anaesthetists examined anaesthetic related deaths. During the following five years over 1000 deaths were voluntarily reported by anaesthetists; anaesthesia contributed to 59 per cent of deaths. The commonest causes were aspiration of gastric contents and relative overdose of barbiturates. The Report on Confidential Enquiries into maternal deaths has appeared triennially for over thirty years. Between 1991 and 1995, there were 9.8 deaths per 100,000 maternities, with 228 deaths related to anaesthesia. Substandard care was implicated in seven of the eight direct anaesthetic fatalities. Hypoxaemia and airway obstruction were still leading causes of death. This report resulted in evaluation of anaesthetic services for maternity units and has encouraged the appraisal of standards of care. In 1982 Lunn and Mushin studied mortality in patients dying within six days of surgery in six regions in Great Britain. The study included 1.1 million anaesthetics, and reported 6060 deaths. Slightly fewer than 10 per cent of deaths were influenced by anaesthesia, and more than 50 per cent of deaths occurred in the over 70 age group. It was realized that both anaesthetists and surgeons should be involved in the evaluation of postoperative deaths. In 1986 a joint working party of the Associations of Anaesthetists and Surgeons organized a National Confidential Enquiry into Perioperative Deaths (NCEPOD). This venture involved co-operation between surgeons and anaesthetists, who considered deaths within 30 days of surgery in three regions. Anaesthesia directly caused one death for every 185 000 operations, and contributed to a further 1300 of the deaths in the study. Deaths were related to inexperienced staff working unsupervized, outside their areas of expertise. The report highlighted the needs to reduce 'out-of-hours work', improve communication between surgeons and anaesthetists, and to keep adequate records. The most recent NCEPOD report recommended more supervision of trainees and increased high dependency and intensive care facilities. It proposed written standards of practice and development of guidelines for good practice.

The causes of anaesthetic related mortality have not changed greatly over the years: they are still hypoxaemia, aspiration of gastric contents, and hypovolaemia. Hypoxaemia due to failure to intubate the trachea or to detect oesophageal intubation can be fatal. Assessment of patients to predict difficult intubation, preoxygenation, adequate trained assistance for the anaesthetist, training in a 'failed intubation drill', availability of aids to intubation, the use of capnography to detect oesophageal intubation, and the use of pulse oximetry are important in the prevention of this complication. Aspiration of gastric contents during induction or recovery causes 20 per cent of perioperative deaths. Patients are particularly at risk after trauma or during pregnancy. Prevention includes reducing the volume of gastric contents and the use of a 'rapid sequence anaesthetic induction' technique. Hypovolaemia is dangerous when combined with the vasodilation of anaesthesia in dehydrated or bleeding patients, who can develop profound and sometimes fatal hypotension. Careful preoperative assessment with resuscitation and adequate monitoring are essential in reducing this complication. A fifth of patients experience problems during the recovery period, and the importance of adequate recovery facilities is emphasized in all mortality reports. The findings of NCEPOD reports will improve the care of patients and suggest minimum standards for anaesthetic monitoring.

Further reading

Associations of Anaesthetists and Surgeons (1996). *Report of the National Confidential Enquiry into Perioperative Deaths 1993/94.* A A G B I, London.

Association of Anaesthetists of Great Britain and Ireland (1988). *Recommendations for standards of monitoring.* A A G B I, London.

Association of Anaesthetists of Great Britain and Ireland (1988). *Assistance for the anaesthetist,* A A G B I, London.

Buck, N., Devlin, H. B., and Lunn, J. W. (1987). *The report of a confidential enquiry into perioperative deaths.* The Nuffield Provincial Hospitals Trust and the Kings Fund, London.

Department of Health and Social Security (1996). *Report on confidential enquiries into maternal deaths in England and Wales 1991–95.* HMSO, London.

Edwards, G., Morton, H. J., Pask, E. A., and Wylie, W. D. (1956). Deaths associated with anaesthesia: a report of 1000 cases. *Anaesthesia,* **11**, 194– 220.

Lunn, J. N. and Mushin, W. W. (1982). *Mortality associated with anaesthesia.* Nuffield Provincial Hospitals Trust, London.

Manninen, P. H. (1991). Anaesthesia outside the operating room. *Canadian Anaesthetists Society Journal,* **38**, R126–9.

Winter, A. and Spence, A. A. (1989). An international consensus on mortality. *British Journal of Anaesthesia,* **64**, 263– 6.

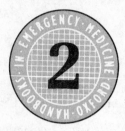

CHAPTER 2

Pharmacology of drugs, gases, and vapours used during general anaesthesia

Key points in pharmacology

- Intravenous anaesthetic induction agents must be given slowly and in reduced doses to shocked or elderly patients to avoid profound cardiorespiratory depression.
- Etomidate has less effect on the cardiovascular system than barbiturates or propofol and may be the drug of choice when cardiovascular stability is needed.
- Nitrous oxide should be avoided if there is air in body cavities, for example a pneumothorax, (unless a chest drain is *in situ*), air embolus, or intracranial air.
- Volatile anaesthesia increases cerebral blood flow and should be avoided if intracranial pressure is elevated.
- The use of naloxone to reverse the effects of opioids at the end of anaesthesia is not recommended.
- Muscle relaxants should not be used at induction if intubation is expected to be difficult.
- Suxamethonium is contraindicated in patients with burns of over 10 per cent, large areas of denervated muscle (paraplegia or crush injury), or raised intraocular or intracranial pressure.

Anticholinergic drugs

Sympathetic and parasympathetic nerve endings are either cholinergic, secreting acetylcholine, or adrenergic, secreting noradrenaline. The preganglionic neurones are all cholinergic, as are postganglionic parasympathetic nerve endings and sympathetic fibres to sweat glands and certain blood vessels. All other postganglionic sympathetic fibres are adrenergic. Ganglionic transmission involves nicotinic cholinergic receptors, and is blocked by ganglion blockers. Postganglionic transmission involves muscarinic cholinergic receptors, and is blocked by atropine and its derivatives.

Indications for anticholinergic drugs

- Premedication to dry secretions for peri-airway surgery.
- Prior to anaesthesia in neonates and small children in some situations.
- Prior to anaesthesia to prevent the vagal effects of certain surgery, for example pulling on extraocular muscles or anal dilatation.
- To prevent bradycardia prior to administering a second dose of suxamethonium.
- To antagonize the muscarinic effects of anticholinesterases such as neostigmine, which are used to reverse muscle relaxants.
- To treat bradycardia once causes such as hypoxaemia have been excluded.

Contraindications to anticholinergic drugs

- Closed angle glaucoma
- Hyoscine may cause confusion in elderly patients

Anticholinergic drugs used for anaesthesia

Atropine

A belladonna alkaloid which crosses the blood–brain barrier, The adult intravenous dose is 0.6 mg and the paediatric dose is 0.02 mg/kg. It produces central nervous system stimulation, but high doses can lead to central depression. It dilates the pupils. Sweating is prevented, and large doses cause a rise in body temperature, especially in children. Atropine peripherally inhibits cardiac vagal activity and increases heart rate; but small doses can lead to a period of bradycardia. It can lead to tachyarrhythmias, which may be dangerous in patients with cardiac problems. It is the anticholinergic drug of choice in the treatment of bradycardia of vagal origin. It is a bronchodilator which reduces and thickens salivary and bronchial secretions. It reduces the volume and acidity of gastric contents, and is antiemetic. It relaxes the gastro-oesophageal sphincter, gut, and ureteric musculature.

Hyoscine hydrobromide
The peripheral effects of hyoscine are qualitatively similar to those of atropine, but hyoscine has more profound central effects, such as sedation and amnesia. The dose of hyoscine is 0.2–0.4 mg intramuscularly in adults. The paediatric dose is 4–8 μg/kg. It may cause confusion in elderly patients. It is a sedative and a more potent antiemetic than atropine. It has a more powerful antisialogogic effect, but less effect on the heart rate than atropine. It relaxes smooth muscle spasm, and is used to treat colicky pain. A transdermal patch has been used to treat motion sickness.

Glycopyrrolate
A quaternary ammonium compound which does not cross the blood–brain barrier. The adult dose is 0.2–0.4 mg intravenously. The paediatric dose is 4–8 μg/kg. It has qualitatively similar peripheral effects to atropine. It has a greater and more prolonged antisialogogic action than atropine or hyoscine. It has less effect on heart rate than atropine, and does not cause tachycardia; it is therefore preferable in patients with cardiac problems. It is less effective than atropine for the treatment of bradycardia. It is longer acting than atropine, and this, together with its cardiac stability, makes it the ideal drug for use with anticholinesterases to reverse neuromuscular blockade.

Intravenous induction agents

An anaesthetic induction agent is rapidly diluted after intravenous administration as it passes through the pulmonary circulation and enters the systemic circulation to reach the target organ, the brain. The dose of drug received by different tissues depends on cardiac output and tissue perfusion. Under normal circumstances the brain, heart, liver, and kidneys receive a higher proportion of the dose of drug than 'vessel-poor' tissues such as skin and muscle. Fat is the least perfused tissue, and receives the smallest dose of drug; but it acts as a drug depot. In low cardiac output states the onset of anaesthesia may be delayed, but the brain receives a higher proportion of the cardiac output, and therefore of the drug. Hypovolaemic patients must be given a reduced dose of intravenous induction agent to prevent profound central nervous and cardiorespiratory depression.

Anaesthetic drugs must be able to enter the brain cells to exert their effect, so they must be lipid soluble and not bound to plasma proteins. Lipid solubility depends on the chemical structure of the drug and its degree of ionization. Highly ionized drugs are not lipid soluble. The high lipid solubility of intravenous induction agents has led to problems with formulation. Most induction agents are highly protein-bound, but rapid intravenous administration saturates binding sites and allows free drug to reach the brain. Initial recovery from anaesthesia depends mainly on redistribution of the drug rather than its elimination.

Drug disposition is usually described using multicompartmental models. Kinetic modelling obviates the need for measurement of tissue drug levels. There may be two or three rates of decline in the plasma concentration of a drug. The initial decay in concentration is rapid, and is due to redistribution into peripheral compartments (alpha phase). The slower decay in concentration is due to drug elimination (beta phase). Half lives for distribution and elimination can be calculated. Volumes of drug distribution can be estimated – the total volume distribution at steady state (V_{dss}) is the mass of drug within the body divided by the plasma drug concentration. This volume may exceed total body water with highly lipid soluble agents. Drugs with a high V_{dss} are freely distributed and bound to tissue proteins, so they do not remain intravascular for long. Plasma clearance is calculated as the volume of plasma which is completely cleared of drug per unit time, and can be separated into renal and extrarenal components. Some drugs are almost completely cleared from the plasma after one passage through the liver, and depend on hepatic blood flow for elimination. Other drugs with a low hepatic extraction ratio are not affected by changes in liver blood flow, but may be cleared by hepatic microsomal enzymes.

A knowledge of kinetic data is useful clinically. Factors which increase the free fraction of the drug may be used to achieve therapeutic rather than toxic drug levels. When using total intravenous anaesthesia, steady-state conditions may be achieved by injecting a bolus of drug and following this by an infusion which is reduced with time. Once steady state has been achieved the rate of infusion should equal the plasma clearance of the drug.

The ideal intravenous induction agent should be water soluble, stable, rapidly acting, and non-irritant to tissues. It should have a high plasma clearance, a high therapeutic index, and a low incidence of predictable or idiosyncratic adverse effects. Analgesic and antiemetic properties would be an advantage. As yet no agent fulfils all these criteria.

Indications for intravenous anaesthetic induction agents

- Induction of anaesthesia
- Sole agent for short procedures, for example cardioversion
- Total intravenous anaesthesia
- Treatment of status epilepticus
- Sedation of a ventilated patient

Contraindications to intravenous anaesthetic induction agents

- Upper airway obstruction
- Unventilated asthmatic
- Severe hypovolaemia
- Known sensitivity to the agent

- Methohexitone should be avoided in epileptics
- Etomidate is not used for long term sedation because of its adrenocortical depressant effects
- Ketamine should not be used in the presence of cardio-vascular disease or raised intracranial or intraocular pressure
- In patients with acute intermittent porphyria, barbiturates are unsafe, etomidate is posssibly unsafe, propofol is possibly safe, and ketamine is contentious.

The pharmacolcinetic properties of each drug are shown in Table 2.1

Barbiturates

Urea and malonic acid combine to form barbituric acid, whose derivatives are commonly used intravenous anaesthetic induction agents. They are the standard against which all other agents are judged.

Thiopentone is a sulphur analogue of pentobarbitone. It needs to be freshly prepared as a 2.5 per cent alkaline solution which is bactericidal. Recovery from a single dose occurs within minutes because of redistribution of the drug from the brain to other 'vessel-rich' tissues such as the liver or kidney. Thiopentone reduces cerebral blood flow, decreases cerebral metabolism, and lowers intracranial pressure; but there is no support for its use as cerebral protection after cardiac arrest or head injury. It is a potent anticonvulsant. Cardiovascular depression is dose related. A normal induction dose in healthy people decreases cardiac output and mean arterial pressure by 20 per cent, and results in a

Table 2.1 • Pharmacokinetic properties of intravenous induction agents

	pH	pK_a	Protein binding (%)	Volume of distribution (l)	Clearance (mg/kg/min)	Elimination half life (h)	Intravenous dose (mg)
Thiopentone	10.5	7.6	80	172	1.4–5.7	5.0–11.6	3.5–5.0
Methohexitone	11.1	7.9	80	168	10–13	1.6–3.9	1–1.5
Etomidate	4.5	4.2	75	380	10–24	1.0–5.4	0.3
Ketamine*	4.5	7.5	20	214	17–20	3.0	1–2*
Propofol	7.4	11	98	771	25–31	11.2	1.5–2.5

*Intramuscular dose 5–10 mg/kg.

compensatory increase in heart rate. Smaller doses and slower administration should be used for patients with reduced cardiac output or myocardial problems. Respiratory depression is also dose related. Thiopentone may increase the irritability of the upper airway, and may provoke bronchopasm. The liver is the main site of metabolism, and 15 per cent of the injected dose is metabolized each hour. The main oxidative metabolites have little hypnotic activity, but prolonged administration may result in the production of hypnotically active pentobarbitone. Only 1 per cent of the dose is renally excreted. The clearance is not altered by changes in liver blood flow. Thiopentone is not suitable for continuous infusion, as it tends to accumulate.

Methohexitone is an oxybarbiturate, with a methyl group which confers convulsant properties and causes excitatory effects during the induction of anaesthesia, for example hiccough and muscle movements. It is contraindicated in epileptics. It needs to be freshly prepared and the solution is alkaline. It can produce pain on injection. The use of 1 ml of 1 per cent plain lignocaine, either given into the vein before injection or mixed with the induction agent, may reduce pain on the injection of methohexitone or other painful induction agents. Injection into a free-running intravenous cannula also reduces pain on injection. Methohexitone is more potent than thiopentone. Methohexitone produces similar central nervous system and cardiorespiratory effects to thiopentone. Full recovery occurs more quickly after methohexitone than after thiopentone.

Etomidate
This imidazole derivative has a structure unlike any other induction agent. It is marketed in propylene glycol. It is more potent than the barbiturates. It is painful on injection, and produces excitatory effects which are myoclonic and not due to a central action. It has less effect on the cardiovascular and respiratory systems than the barbiturates or propofol, and may be the drug of choice when cardiovascular stability is needed. It is rapidly hydrolysed by liver enzymes and plasma esterases (it does not interact with suxamethonium) to inactive metabolites. It has a high hepatic extraction ratio, and its clearance is affected by liver blood flow. Less than 2 per cent of the dose is excreted unchanged by the kidneys.

It depresses adrenocortical function, even in a single dose, and therefore cannot be used for long term sedation.

Ketamine

This phencyclidine derivative produces a slow onset of a dissociated state, and is therefore not really an intravenous induction agent. It produces amnesia and profound analgesia in 2–7 minutes after intravenous injection, but takes twice as long after intramuscular administration. It increases cerebral blood flow and intracranial and intraocular pressures. Emergence is complicated by psychic disturbances, especially in adults. It produces hypertension, and increases myocardial oxygen demand. It should be avoided in patients with cardiovascular disease. It induces salivation, and does not preserve protective reflexes, as was once believed. It has active metabolites and a high hepatic extraction ratio: therefore liver disease has little effect on its metabolism. It may be useful in providing analgesia and a dissociated state in 'field situations', for example at the site of accidents (see p. 90).

Propofol

This alkyl phenol is marketed in soya bean oil and egg phosphatide. The formulation supports the growth of bacteria and yeasts, so care must be taken with sterility once the ampoule is opened. It produces pain on injection which may be reduced by the prior use of lignocaine or alfentanil. It produces rapid induction and recovery with a reduced incidence of nausea and vomiting. It causes a greater fall in blood pressure than the barbiturates, and should be used with caution in elderly or hypovolaemic patients, when the dose must be reduced. It depresses laryngeal reflexes more than the barbiturates, It is useful as an infusion for total intravenous anaesthesia as it does not accumulate. A possible regimen to follow induction of anaesthesia would be 10 mg/kg/h for 15 min, 8 mg/kg/h for 15 min, and then 6 mg/kg/h. If anaesthesia is too light, a bolus of 0.5 mg/kg may be used, which can be repeated if necessary after 15 min, then the infusion should be increased by 2 mg/kg/h. If anaesthesia is too deep, the infusion should be reduced by 2 mg/kg/h. Propofol can be used to provide sedation for minor procedures under local anaesthesia, either by infusion or patient controlled pump.

Inhalational anaesthesia gases and vapours

The physico-chemical properties of inhalational anaesthetic agents determine their potency, rate of uptake, and speed of elimination (Table 2.2). The potency reflects the ability to achieve anaesthesia at a steady-state inspired concentration, and depends on the oil:gas partition coefficient of the agent. Potent drugs are highly oil soluble. The concept of minimum alveolar concentration (MAC) allows comparison of the potency of different agents. The MAC is defined as the alveolar concentration of an agent, in air at one atmosphere, needed to abolish movement in response to a surgical stimulus in 50 per cent of patients. The MAC is measured after a period of equilibration, as the concept assumes that the brain, arterial blood, alveolar, and end tidal concentrations are in equilibrium.

The blood:gas partition coefficient determines the rapidity of induction of and recovery from anaesthesia. Agents with a low blood solubility, such as isoflurane, produce rapid induction and recovery, and allow the depth of anaesthesia to be adjusted quickly. The potency of the drug must also be taken into account, and nitrous oxide (MAC 105) is not a potent agent when compared with halothane (MAC 0.75).

Ideal inhalational agents must be capable of being produced in a pure form relatively cheaply. They should be stable in light and in the presence of soda lime. They must not be flammable in the presence of air, oxygen, or nitrous

Table 2.2 • Physicochemical properties of anaesthetic gases and vapours

	Boiling point (°C)	SVP (%)	Partition coefficients		MAC (%)	Metabolized (%)
			Oil:gas	Blood:gas		
Nitrous oxide	−89	–	1.4	0.47	105	–
Halothane	50	33	244	2.3	0.75	46
Enflurane	56	24	96	1.9	1.68	8.5
Isoflurane	48	33	91	1.4	1.15	0.2
Desflurane	23	88	18.7	0.42	6.0	0.02
Sevoflurane	55	24	42	0.68	1.71	2

SVP (saturated vapour pressure)

oxide – therefore agents such as ether and cyclopropane are no longer used. Inhalational agents should be non-irritant, free from adverse cardiorespiratory effects, and analgesic. A good inhalational agent is not extensively metabolized, and is therefore less likely to produce reactive metabolites, free radicals, or inorganic fluoride, which might result in organ toxicity. Isoflurane is superior to halothane in this respect. As yet no agent fulfils all the ideals.

Indications for inhalational agents

- Induction of anaesthesia. Gaseous induction is preferred by some children. Although gaseous induction is more difficult in adults it may be needed in cases of upper airway problems.
- Maintenance of anaesthesia.
- To provide analgesia, for example Entonox (see p. 23 and 233).
- Sedation during procedures under local anaesthesia.

Contraindications to inhalational agents

- Nitrous oxide should be avoided in the presence of air in body cavities – for example in cases of pneumothorax (unless a chest drain is *in situ*), air embolus, or intracranial air.
- Some volatile anaesthetic agents increase cerebral blood flow, and should be avoided in the presence of raised intracranial pressure, for example halothane and desflurane. Low concentrations of isoflurane and sevoflurane may be used with care in patients with high intracranial pressure.
- Nitrous oxide in concentrations in excess of 50 per cent and all volatile agents are contraindicated in patients susceptible to malignant hyperthermia.
- The risk of hepatitis contraindicates repeated use of halothane within three months and its use in patients with a history of unexplained jaundice or pyrexia after previous halothane exposure.
- Enflurane is contraindicated in epilepsy.

Gases used in anaesthesia

Oxygen

This forms 20.95 per cent of the atmosphere, and is very chemically reactive. It supports combustion, so that substances will burn more vigorously, and may explode, when ignited in oxygen. Oxygen is a drug which must be administered in a controlled manner. 100 per cent oxygen should always be used in patients suffering cardiorespiratory arrest, and in shock. Administration of high concentrations of oxygen to spontaneously breathing patients with chronic chest problems may compromise ventilation due to suppression of hypoxic drive. When the concentration of inspired oxygen is important, Venturi masks must be used to deliver predictable concentrations. Long term ventilation with high oxygen concentrations can lead to blindness in neonates and lung damage in adults and children; but this is not a consideration in the A & E setting.

Nitrous oxide

This is a non-irritant, sweet smelling gas which is heavier than air. It is neither flammable nor explosive, but will support the combustion of other agents, even in the absence of oxygen. Nitrous oxide has a low blood–gas partition coefficient, and is rapidly absorbed from the lungs. It is analgesic in an inspired concentration of 50 per cent, but it is not a potent anaesthetic. It has a MAC of 105, and cannot produce anaesthesia when used alone, unless it is given in a concentration which results in hypoxaemia. Nitrous oxide reduces the MAC of other inhalational agents. It can cause cardiovascular depression in some patients. It is 15 times more soluble in plasma than nitrogen, and 100 times more soluble than oxygen. It replaces nitrogen in any body cavity, and can cause an increase in pressure in the middle ear or expand a pneumothorax or intracranial air. It diffuses into the gut during surgery, and may compromise anastomotic healing and delay the return of bowel function. It rapidly diffuses into the lungs at the end of anaesthesia and may result in hypoxaemia; therefore 100 per cent oxygen is usually administered at the end of an anaesthetic. Long term use of nitrous oxide for 6–12 hours can produce bone marrow problems by oxidizing vitamin B12. Chronic exposure has been associated with megaloblastic anaemia with neurological defects.

Entonox

The addition of oxygen to nitrous oxide lowers its critical temperature until, at a 50 per cent mixture, it can be stored as a compressed gas. If Entonox cylinders are exposed to low environmental temperatures the oxygen and nitrous oxide may separate, giving the potential for delivery of a hypoxic mixture. Entonox is an effective analgesic, which can be used safely by non-medical personnel using a demand valve system. It needs to be inhaled for 45 seconds before the maximum analgesic effect is achieved. Once inhalation ceases the alveolar concentration falls quickly, and analgesia is short lived.

Air

Concerns about the adverse effects of nitrous oxide and atmospheric pollution have resulted in air being used more frequently during anaesthesia. Medical air is supplied from cylinders or pipelines. It can be used to nebulize salbutamol or ipratropium bromide if high inspired oxygen concentrations are undesirable.

Carbon dioxide

This is a colourless gas which is present as 0.03 per cent of the atmosphere. It is irritant to the mucosa when inhaled in high concentration. There have been reports of high concentrations of carbon dioxide being administered accidentally. It is recommended that carbon dioxide is not routinely kept on anaesthetic machines.

Volatile anaesthetic agents

Halothane

This is a halogenated hydrocarbon which is non-flammable in anaesthetic concentrations at one atmosphere. It can be broken down by light, and is therefore stored in brown bottles with 0.01 per cent thymol as a stabilizer. It is a potent agent, with marked cardiovascular effects. It produces a dose-related reduction in myocardial contractility, cardiac output, and mean arterial blood pressure. The heart rate tends to fall because of a direct effect on the conducting system, and arrhythmias are common. It has little direct effect on coronary arteries. It sensitizes the heart to endogenous and exogenous catecholamines, especially in the presence of hypercapnia. Adrenaline should not be administered to patients breathing halothane. It is a respiratory depressant, and decreases the normal response to hypoxia and hypercapnia. It is a bronchodilator. It increases cerebral blood flow and reduces splanchnic, renal, and liver blood flows. It potentiates the effects of muscle relaxants. It produces uterine relaxation. Halothane is not an analgesic agent.

Rarely, a serious fulminant hepatic failure can follow halothane anaesthesia. The diagnosis can be confirmed serologically in both adults and children by showing *in vitro* serum antibodies reacting with halothane-altered liver cell membrane determinants. It occurs more often after repeated exposure to halothane, and has a high mortality. Halothane is normally metabolized by oxidation to several products, such as trifluoroacetic acid, chloride, and bromide. It is thought that halothane hepatitis may be caused by halothane metabolites reacting with hepatic macromolecules to produce liver damage. Therefore enzyme induction and liver hypoxia may be predisposing factors. Obesity, leading to a storage of halothane in the fat, may also be important.

Enflurane

This is a stable, non-flammable ether stored without a preservative. Its blood solubility and cardiovascular effects fall between those of halothane and isoflurane. It reduces myocardial contractility, cardiac output, and mean arterial blood pressure to a lesser extent than halothane, and more than isoflurane. Unlike halothane it decreases systemic vascular resistance. It is less arrhythmogenic, and sensitizes the myocardium to catecholamines less than halothane. It decreases coronary artery resistance, but less so than isoflurane. It is more respiratory depressant than either halothane or isoflurane, and is a bronchodilator. It can produce generalized convulsions, and is therefore contraindicated in epileptics. It increases cerebral blood flow and reduces renal blood flow. The plasma fluoride concentration is greater after enflurane anaesthesia than after halothane or isoflurane; but the concentration reached is below that needed to produce renal toxicity, and is not influenced by enzyme induction. It may be sensible to avoid prolonged use of enflurane in patients with renal failure. Enflurane potentiates the effects of muscle relaxants more than halothane or isoflurane; but it relaxes the uterus in a similar manner. Although ethers are more analgesic than hydrocarbons, enflurane is rapidly eliminated, and does not seem to contribute much to postoperative pain relief. Enflurane is metabolized less extensively, and has a smaller effect on liver blood flow than halothane. Enflurane is therefore potentially less toxic than halothane.

Isoflurane
This is a structural isomer of enflurane, but is more difficult to prepare and more expensive. It is non-flammable, stable, and needs no preservative. It is possible to adjust the level of anaesthesia more quickly with isoflurane, as it is less soluble in blood than halothane or enflurane. Isoflurane has less effect on myocardial contractility and cardiac output than enflurane or halothane. It decreases arterial blood pressure because it reduces systemic vascular resistance. Isoflurane is a coronary vasodilator, but redistribution of coronary blood flow may cause ischaemia in patients with multiple vessel coronary artery disease. It does not commonly cause arrhythmias, and does not sensitize the heart to catecholamines. It is more of a respiratory depressant than halothane, and less of a respiratory depressant than enflurane. It is a bronchodilator. It has no convulsive effects, and less than 1.0 MAC of isoflurane does not alter cerebral blood flow if the patient is normocapnic. Isoflurane does not affect liver or renal blood flow as much as the other agents. The potential for renal toxicity is negligible. It potentiates muscle relaxants, as do all ethers. Its metabolism is minimal, which greatly reduces its potential for organ toxicity.

Desflurane
This is a fluorinated analogue of isoflurane. It is non-flammable, stable, and needs no preservative. It has to be administered through a modified vaporizer because of its low boiling point. The vaporizers are electrically heated and pressurized. It has a very low blood gas solubility, so that induction of anaesthesia, adjustment of the depth of anaesthesia, and recovery are rapid. Its pungency limits its use for gaseous induction. Its cardiovascular safety is greater than that of halothane and enflurane, but not as great as that of

isoflurane. Desflurane does not lead to arrhythmias or sensitize the heart to catecholamines. It produces less coronary vasodilation than isoflurane or sevoflurane. Desflurane produces respiratory depression intermediate between enflurane and isoflurane. It is a cerebral vasodilator. This effect outweighs its effect to reduce cerebral metabolism. It therefore increases intracranial pressure. It is not metabolized significantly and therefore has a low propensity for organ toxicity.

Sevoflurane

This is a fluorinated ether. It is non-flammable and requires no preservative. It is broken down in soda lime (calcium oxide with sodium hydroxide) in a temperature dependent manner (6.5 per cent per hour at 20°C and 57 per cent per hour at 54°C) to form 'compound A' (breakdown is greater in Baralyme). The clinical significance of this is uncertain. It has a low blood gas solubility resulting in rapid induction and recovery, which is not quite as fast as with desflurane but faster than with isoflurane. Sevoflurane is non-pungent and good for inhalational induction. It reduces blood pressure less than does isoflurane. It does not cause cardiac arrhythmias or sensitize the myocardium to catecholamines. It is less respiratory depressant than desflurane, isoflurane, and enflurane, but more than halothane. Sevoflurane is similar to isoflurane in its clinically insignificant effect on intracranial pressure. Biotransformation to inorganic fluoride is greater than with enflurane. The rapid elimination of sevoflurane from the lung may mean that less is available for biotransformation after the cessation of inhalation. This may reduce the risk of renal toxicity after use of sevoflurane.

Analgesics (see p. 237)

Potent intravenous opioids are used during the induction and maintenance of anaesthesia, and to provide initial postoperative analgesia. Short acting drugs such as fentanyl and alfentanil are commonly employed. The use of naloxone to reverse the effects of these agents at the end of anaesthesia is not recommended, as it may produce hypertension, pulmonary oedema, or cardiac arrest, and its duration does not always outlast that of the opioid.

Respiratory stimulants

Doxapram acts directly on the medulla to stimulate breathing. There are few indications for the use of these agents in modern anaesthesia. There may be a place for cautious use in selected patients with chest problems to facilitate recovery from anaesthesia. Doxapram has also been used in the treatment of buprenorphine overdose.

Muscle relaxants

A nerve impulse causes acetylcholine to be released at the neuromuscular junction (NMJ). Acetylcholine binds with nicotinic receptors on the postjunctional membrane and opens ion channels, depolarizing the end-plate and triggering muscle contraction, which involves calcium. Acetylcholinesterase is an enzyme which is stored close to the receptor membrane. It breaks down acetylcholine, and results in repolarization of the end-plate membrane before the next impulse. Prejunctional receptors are involved in feedback control mechanisms at the NMJ.

Neuromuscular transmission may be interrupted by drugs which block acetylcholine synthesis (hemicholinium) or release (aminoglycoside antibiotics). Drugs which combine with acetylcholine receptors are commonly termed neuromuscular blockers. There are two types: depolarizing, for example suxamethonium, and non-depolarizing, for example atracurium.

Indications for muscle relaxants

- To permit intubation
- To allow ventilation
- To facilitate surgery

Contraindications to muscle relaxants

- Where intubation is suspected or known to be difficult.
- Care in patients with neuromuscular diseases, for example myasthenia gravis or myotonia.
- In patients with acute intermittent porphyria, suxamethonium is safe, vecuronium is possibly safe, pancuronium is contentious and there are few data available about other relaxants.

Muscle relaxants used for anaesthesia

Suxamethonium

This depolarizing neuromuscular blocker has a structure which resembles two linked acetylcholine molecules. It hydrolyses slowly at room temperature, and should be stored in the refrigerator. The intravenous dose is 1.0 mg/kg, which acts within 30 seconds to produce fasciculations and then flaccid paralysis. A higher dose may be needed in neonates. No other drug produces total paralysis as quickly. It remains the agent of choice for rapid sequence induction of anaesthesia. It can be given intramuscularly in a dose of 2 mg/kg, but the onset takes 3–4 minutes. It raises intra-ocular and intracranial pressures. It increases the plasma potassium concentration. It has muscarinic effects, such as bradycardia (especially after a second dose), salivation, and an increase in bronchial secretions. Its duration of action is about five minutes. Hydrolysis by plasma cholinesterase terminates its effect. Some individuals have a genetically determined abnormality of this enzyme that prolongs the effect of suxamethonium and results in apnoea. Liver disease, organophosphorus agents, and plasmapheresis all augment the effect of suxamethonium. Muscular pains (scoline pains) commonly occur after its use. These are a particular problem in young patients who are quickly ambulant after surgery.

Contraindications to suxamethonium
- Hyperkalaemia.
- Patients with more than 10 per cent burns may sustain a fatal increase in plasma potassium if suxamethonium is given 5–120 days after the burn.

- Dangerous rises in plasma potassium may occur during a similar period in patients with large areas of denervated muscle, as for example in paraplegia or crush injury.
- Suxamethonium has an unpredictable effect in the presence of chronic wasting muscle diseases.
- Raised intraocular or intracranial pressure.
- Plasma cholinesterase abnormality.
- Susceptibility to malignant hyperthermia.

Non-depolarizing muscle relaxants
All the clinically useful agents are quaternary ammonium compounds, which are ionized at body pH. They are not lipid soluble, and do not cross the blood–brain barrier or placenta easily. The ideal neuromuscular blocker should be non-depolarizing, to avoid the unwanted effects of increased muscle tone, such as raised intraocular pressure and pain. It should have rapid onset, be easily reversible within 10 minutes of administration, and non-cumulative after repeated doses. It should be specific for the NMJ, to avoid cardiovascular and other muscarinic side-effects. It should not release histamine. Newer agents fulfil these criteria better than the older drugs such as tubocurarine and pancuronium.

Atracurium besylate
This bisquaternary ammonium compound is presented in an aqueous solution, which should be kept at 4°C. It is denatured by alkali. If dilution is necessary, it should be mixed with normal saline, not water. The paralysing dose is 0.4–0.6 mg/kg, which takes 90 seconds to be effective. Atracurium causes local histamine release, but allergic reactions are rare. Paralysis can be maintained by infusion of a dose equivalent to the induction dose each hour, using NMJ monitoring to adjust the rate. It is specific for the NMJ, and has no muscarinic actions at normal doses. It is broken down in the plasma by spontaneous ester hydrolysis and Hofmann elimination. It does not accumulate, and reversal is easy and complete. It is ideal for patients with hepatic or renal disease, as it does not rely on enzymatic degradation or renal clearance for elimination. Concern has been expressed about the central nervous effects of its breakdown product laudanosine; however, problems are more likely during

prolonged infusion in Intensive Care Units in patients with poor renal function.

Vecuronium
This is a monoquaternary ammonium steroidal compound. The paralysing dose is 0.1 mg/kg, which takes 90–120 seconds to take full effect. Paralysis may be maintained by the use of an infusion of 0.08 mg/kg/h. Vecuronium does not release histamine. It is specific for the NMJ, and has no muscarinic actions at normal doses. Cumulation is minimal after repeated doses. It is rapidly cleared from plasma by distribution to the liver, where it is metabolized. 20 per cent of the dose is excreted renally and 12 per cent is excreted in bile during the first 24 hours. It should be used with caution in patients with renal impairment.

Mivacurium
This monoquaternary compound is presented as a mixture of cis–trans isomers. It is less potent than vecuronium; the adult intubating dose is 0.15 mg/kg. Children may need a relatively larger dose. Large doses may cause histamine release. It has a rapid onset, but is not as fast as suxamethonium, which it cannot replace. Its duration of action is about half that of atracurium. It may be used as an infusion (0.6 mg/kg/h). It is rapidly broken down by plasma cholinesterase to inactive products. Patients with abnormalities of cholinesterase may show a change in duration of action of mivacurium. It is also eliminated by the liver and kidney. The duration of block is increased 1.5-fold in renal failure and three-fold in hepatic failure.

Rocuronium
This monoquarternay aminosteroidal neuromuscular blocker is about one seventh as potent as vecuronium. It has a faster onset and an intermediate duration of action. The dose is 0.45–0.6 mg/kg. Its propensity to release histamine is negligible. It has minimal cardiovascular effects. Its plasma clearance is mainly due to liver uptake and biliary excretion. Its duration of action may be increased in those with hepatic or renal problems.

Cisatracurium
This is a purified form of one of the ten isomers of atracurium. It is three times more potent than atracurium. The

dose is 0.1 mg/kg. It has a slightly slower onset than atracurium, but spontaneous recovery occurs at about the same rate. It is less likely to release histamine than atracurium. It is predominantly eliminated by Hofmann degredation and does not accumulate in patients with renal or hepatic problems.

Reversal of neuromuscular blockade
Non-depolarizing neuromuscular block can be antagonized by increasing the concentration of acetylcholine at the NMJ using anticholinesterase drugs such as neostigmine. The dose of neostigmine is 2.5–5.0 mg in an adult. Anti-muscarinic agents must be given simultaneously to avoid the cardiac and other side effects. The usual combination is with 0.5 mg glycopyrrolate for each 2.5 mg of neostigmine. Large doses of neostigmine or its use in the absence of non-depolarizing blockers may cause paralysis.

Factors which potentiate non-depolarizing neuromuscular block
- Hyperventilation
- Ether anaesthetics
- Hypothermia
- Acidosis
- Aminoglycoside antibiotics
- Muscle diseases
- Overdose of anticholinesterase drugs

Factors which lead to resistance to non-depolarizing neuromuscular block
- Increased acute phase proteins
- Altered volume distribution in hepatic or renal disease
- Increased number of receptor sites, for example, in hemiplegia, multiple sclerosis, or disuse muscle atrophy

Further reading

Calvey, T. N. and Williams, N. E. (1991). *Principles and practice of pharmacology for anaesthetists*, (2nd edn). Blackwell Scientific, Oxford.

Hull, C. J. (1991). *Pharmacokinetics for anaesthetists*, Butterworth-Heinemann, Oxford.

Kaufman, L. and Taberner, P. V. (1996). *Pharmacology in the practice of anaesthesia*, Arnold, London.

Vickers, M. D., Morgan, M and Spencer, P. S. J. (1991). *Drugs in anaesthetic practice*. Butterworth-Heinemann, Oxford.

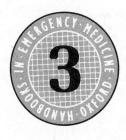

CHAPTER 3

Anaesthetic and resuscitation equipment

Key points in anaesthetic and resuscitation equipment

- All doctors should be familiar with the anaesthetic and resuscitation equipment in their hospital.
- Always check equipment before it is used. Anaesthetic problems are often caused by equipment failures.
- Never bypass safety procedures, no matter how urgent the situation.

Anaesthetic equipment and techniques are continuously changing to provide safer and more efficient anaesthesia. These changes often occur more quickly in the operating theatres than in A & E departments. It is essential, when starting a new job, that each doctor becomes familiar with the resuscitation and anaesthetic equipment used in the hospital.

Gas supply

Cylinders

Medical gases are stored under pressure in metal cylinders. The cylinders are colour coded for each individual gas (Table 3.1). A valve connects the cylinder to the anaesthetic machine or flowmeter. It is opened using a key. The valve is screwed into the cylinder neck. There are two types of valve,

Table 3.1 • Medical gases commonly used in an A & E department

| Gas | ISO and UK coding | | Physical state |
	Cylinder	Cylinder shoulder	
Oxygen	Black	White	Gas
Nitrous oxide	Blue	Blue	Liquid
Air	Grey	White/Black	Gas
Entonox	Blue	White/Blue	Gas

bull-nosed and pin-index. The latter was designed to prevent accidental fitting of the wrong cylinder to the anaesthetic machine. Each gas has a unique pattern of holes on its valve, which coincide with the pins on the appropriate yoke of the anaesthetic machine. The valve is the weakest part of the cylinder, and can be damaged if the cylinder is dropped. A protective cap or plastic sheath often covers the valve outlet to prevent dirt accumulating.

Practical points
- A circular or hexagonal coloured washer at the base of the valve carries the 'test date'. The date of filling is also indicated. If these are not clear or there is any doubt use a different cylinder and send the original back to the suppliers.
- Different keys are required depending on the type of valve. It is important to ensure that each anaesthetic machine has the correct key attached to it.
- Always open cylinder valves slowly. A sudden surge of oxygen in the presence of grease may cause an explosion.
- Always open the valve of a new cylinder for a few seconds to clear away any dirt before attaching it to an anaesthetic machine.
- Leaks usually occur when the valve has not been fully turned off. Alternatively the valve gland may be loose. This can be corrected by tightening the gland nut at the top of the valve stem until the leak just stops.
- Leaks occurring when a pin-index cylinder is connected may indicate the need to replace the sealing washer.

Gas pipelines

Medical gases are supplied by pipeline from large central stores. This is more economical, and removes the need for frequent changing of cylinders. The usual hospital medical gas pipeline pressure is 60 p.s.i. (414 kPa). The outlets and pipe extensions are colour-coded (Table 3.2). Each gas pipeline has a non-interchangeable connection. The pipelines are fitted with isolating taps and warning devices to indicate a reduction in pipeline pressure.

Practical points

- Very rarely hose connections may accidently be crossed over. Daily checks of pipeline function should always be made (see p. 61).

- Full oxygen cylinders must always be available, even when pipelines are in use.

Pressure regulators

The cylinder valve is connected to a pressure regulator, which is necessary to provide a controlled, steady flow of gas. The regulator reduces the gas pressure from cylinder pressure to 60 p.s.i. (414 kPa) thus protecting the anaesthetic apparatus and the patient from dangerously high pressures. The regulator also compensates for any reduction in cylinder pressure as the cylinder empties. Regulators usually have a safety valve. A demand regulator provides a steady flow of gas only when the patient inhales, and is used with Entonox cylinders.

Pressure gauges

A pressure gauge is connected to the inlet of the pressure regulator to indicate when the cylinder is becoming empty.

Table 3.2 • Coding for medical gas pipes, joints, and terminations

Gas	Colour code
Oxygen	White
Nitrous oxide	Blue
Medical air	Black/White
Entonox	Blue/White
Suction	Yellow

Compressed gases, for example oxygen or air, approximately obey the ideal gas law, which means that a fall in volume will produce a proportional fall in pressure. Thus when the cylinder pressure drops to half, it will be about half full. With liquefied gases such as nitrous oxide, the pressure gauge measures saturated vapour pressure. While some liquefied gas remains in the cylinder the gauge will give a constant reading of the saturated vapour pressure, assuming that the temperature remains constant. When the cylinder is about one-quarter full, all the nitrous oxide will be gaseous, and the pressure gauge reading will begin to fall. The weight of the cylinder is the only guide to the amount of nitrous oxide remaining.

Practical points

- Oxygen cylinders are filled to 2000 p.s.i. (13.8 Mpa) and should always be changed when the pointer enters the red zone.
- Nitrous oxide cylinders are filled to 750 p.s.i. (5 Mpa) and should always be changed when the reading enters the red zone.
- Always ensure that the cylinder valve is closed before changing cylinders.
- Residual gas in the pressure gauge may give a positive reading even when the cylinder is turned off. If a cylinder is to be used, always check that the cylinder valve is turned on.

Flowmeters

Flowmeters measure the flow of gas delivered to the patient. They are calibrated in litres/minute. They are connected distal to the pressure regulator on cylinders and anaesthetic machines, and may be wall-mounted. 'Bobbin-type' flowmeters should be read from the top of the float, and 'ball-type' are read from the centre. Inaccuracies may occur if the flowmeter tube is not vertical, if the float sticks because of static electricity or dirt, or if the tube is leaking.

Practical points

- Always turn the rotameters off when the gases are no longer needed. It is wasteful and dangerous to leave flow meters on unnecessarily.

- If the flowmeter reading falls unexpectedly check the gas supply immediately.

Anaesthetic machines

Anaesthetic machine design is continuously changing. There may be many different types within one hospital, and it is the doctor's responsibility to become familiar with their use.

The cylinder yokes carry the pin index and attach the cylinders to the anaesthetic machine. The back bar supports the flowmeters and vaporizers. At one end there is a valve which directs the gas to the outlet or to a circle absorber. All anaesthetic machines are fitted with a pressure relief valve distal to the flowmeters and vaporizers, to protect the machine from high back-pressure. Other safety features include a flowmeter bypass valve for an emergency oxygen supply and an oxygen failure warning device.

Practical points
- If gas is not coming out of the outlet, check that the gas supply is connected and the flowmeters are turned on.
- Always check that the oxygen failure warning device is functioning before commencing anaesthesia.

Vaporizers

Vaporizers introduce controlled concentrations of volatile anaesthetic agents into the anaesthetic gases. Temperature-compensated vaporizers are standard. The required vapour concentration can be set manually, and is maintained over a wide range of temperature changes and gas flows. Each vaporizer should only be used for one particular volatile anaesthetic. A pin-safety system has been developed to prevent accidental filling of a vaporizer with the wrong anaesthetic agent.

Practical points
- Always ensure that the vaporizer is switched off after use.
- Vaporizers should be filled using a closed system to reduce pollution.

- Cross-contamination may occur with vaporizers in series on older machines. This can be prevented by designs placing them in parallel systems. Some anaesthetic machines have a mechanism which prevents two vaporizers being turned on simultaneously.

Oxygen flush (bypass)

This may be situated at the end of the back bar or at the machine outlet. It provides a high flow of oxygen, at least 35 litres/minute, at a pressure of 60 p.s.i. (414 kPa). It is commonly activated by pressing a button, which can be locked on by turning it. The oxygen flush can be used in an emergency when a hypoxaemic patient requires a rapid increase in inspired oxygen concentration. It is also a convenient way of clearing and filling an anaesthetic circuit for pre-oxygenation.

Practical points
- Leaks around the mask may lead to inefficient bag–valve–mask ventilation during resuscitation. In these situations the rebreathing bag does not fill adequately, and it is tempting to maintain the necessary high gas flow by leaving the oxygen flush permanently on. This technique is potentially hazardous. If the patient is intubated and connected to the anaesthetic circuit with the oxygen flush still on, high pressures may be directed to the lungs, causing barotrauma. The oxygen flush must not be used as a substitute for poor technique.
- Flowmeters do not indicate if the oxygen flush is turned on during anaesthesia. Always ensure it is turned off after use. If it is inadvertently left on the patient may not be adequately anaesthetized as a result of dilution of the anaesthetic gases by oxygen.

Other features

Suction units are commonly attached to anaesthetic machines. They usually work from a central suction supply, colour coded yellow. They must be checked before commencing anaesthesia.

Anaesthetic breathing systems

Anaesthetic tubes

Disposable plastic tubing is now in routine use. The tubing must have sufficient diameter to cause minimal resistance to gas flow, and must be of uniform cross-section to promote laminar flow. It must be flexible to prevent kinking.

Practical points
- The tubing corrugations allow acute angulation without kinking, but may cause turbulence and harbour dirt and infection.
- Coaxial circuits have an inner tube running within an outer tube, increasing the risk of kinking or disconnection.

Reservoir bags

These are made of antistatic rubber. A 2.0 litre bag is commonly used for adults, and 500 ml bags are used for children. The bags may have different sizes and designs of neck, requiring care with the choice of connector. Paediatric bags often have an open tail, which is occluded manually during ventilation.

Practical points
- Ageing and inappropriate use may stiffen the bag walls, producing too great a resistance for breathing. Sometimes the walls stick together. Holes may occur in the newest-looking bag. Always check the bag before use.
- The bag should have a capacity greater than the required tidal volume.

Expiratory ('pop-off' or adjustable pressure-limiting) valves

This type of valve allows expired and surplus gas to escape from the breathing circuit. It prevents the entry of gas from outside the system even if there is a negative pressure within the system. However, it must provide sufficient resistance to prevent the reservoir bag from emptying spontaneously, particularly when a scavenging system is used which exerts a sub-atmospheric pressure on it. A commonly used type is the Heidbrink valve. The valve is adjusted by turning the screw top.

Practical points

- Expiratory valves are a major pressure safety device in a breathing system. They are designed to blow off at 70 cm water even if they are screwed down. Older designs tend to stick if dirty, moist, damaged, or aged. The screw top may be difficult to move. Always check the valve before use. Barotrauma may occur if an intubated patient is attached to a system with a closed, stuck expiratory valve. If there is a build-up of pressure in the system and the valve will not open adequately, disconnect the system at the catheter mount to release the pressure, and then release the valve, or, preferably, change to a safe system. Maintain oxygenation of the patient at all times.

- Expiratory valves are delicate. Treat them gently and never leave them fully closed after use.

- The required degree of opening of the valve is different for each patient. It forms part of a balance between the delivered gas flow and the patient's tidal volume and respiratory rate. It can be determined by careful observation of the patient and the anaesthetic system in conjunction with fine alteration of the valve.

- Paediatric systems are usually designed to be valveless, to reduce the resistance to breathing.

Connectors

Catheter mount
This connects the distal end of an anaesthetic system to a tracheal tube. It is made of narrow gauge corrugated or non-corrugated tubing. The upstream end fits to the anaesthetic system by a female tapered connector. The downstream end may have one piece of a two-part tracheal connector, or may slip directly over the tracheal tube connector.

Practical points

- The catheter mount lies downstream to the expiratory valve and thus increases the effective dead space. Catheter mounts must be used with caution in paediatric systems, where too great an increase in dead space may lead to carbon dioxide retention.

- There is a great variety of tracheal connectors. Always ensure the correct ones are available before starting a procedure.

Feed mount
This attaches to the outlet of an anaesthetic machine. Oxygen tubing may be connected at its other end to deliver gas to a self-inflating bag.

Face masks

These are designed to fit the patient's face without any leaks. They should exert minimal pressure to avoid depressing the jaw, causing respiratory obstruction, or producing pressure sores. They are made of rubber, neoprene, or plastic. The transparent types are useful in resuscitation, since they allow early detection of vomit. The edge of the face mask may be fitted with a rolled edge or cuff. The latter is inflated using a small delivery tube and plug situated at the nasal end of the mask. Adult face masks are anatomically shaped, and have a taper at the nasal end. Child and infant masks also have this design. For babies, circular masks with a soft seal fitting over nose and mouth are used.

Practical points
- Various shapes and sizes of mask are available. It is wise to have a selection ready for any one patient, since no two faces are the same.
- The face mask increases the effective dead space. This may be critical in paediatric practice. The smallest face mask does not necessarily give the smallest dead space.
- Ageing or misuse may cause the cuff to puncture. The filling tubes sometimes collapse and stick together, or the plug may be stuck or absent. On some masks, such as the Laerdal, the cuff is held on with bungs, which may be missing, leaving holes through which gas leaks. Check the face mask before use.

Breathing filters

A breathing filter should be placed between the distal end of the anaesthetic system and the face mask or catheter mount in order to keep the anaesthetic tubing, valve, and reservoir bag clean. Breathing filters should provide the maximum filtering of expired gases, but minimum resistance to breathing. The use of filters helps to maintain the humidity of inspired gases. In modern anaesthesia each patient must have a sterile tracheal tube and catheter mount or a clean face mask attached to an uncontaminated breathing system. The use of breathing filters removes the need to change and sterilize the breathing system for each patient. Breathing systems are usually changed each day.

Manual resuscitators (self-inflating bags)

These are most appropriate for resuscitation, particularly when used by those with limited anaesthetic training. Manual resuscitators have three important features. The self-refilling bag needs no fresh gas flow. It can entrain air and is thus invaluable for use outside hospital. Oxygen supplements can be added to enable high concentrations of oxygen to be given to patients, whether they are breathing spontaneously or being ventilated. The one-way valve prevents expired gas mixing with the inspired gas in the bag, thus providing a non-rebreathing system. Refinements such as safety pressure valves and reservoirs are available. Ideal criteria have been laid down for manual resuscitators used in resuscitation (European Resuscitation Council 1996).

There are many different designs. The salient features will be described with reference to the Laerdal silicone resuscitator (Fig. 3.1). This comes in three different sizes, adult, child (7 to 30 kg), and infant (under 7 kg). They are made up of five main parts.

1. **Face masks:** These are transparent, allowing early detection of vomit. The adult and paediatric masks have a cuffed edge, and the connector fits over the connector of the patient valve. The infant face masks are circular and have a rolled edge. The connector of the smaller sizes fits inside the patient valve connector.

2. **Non-rebreathing patient valve:** This allows the venting

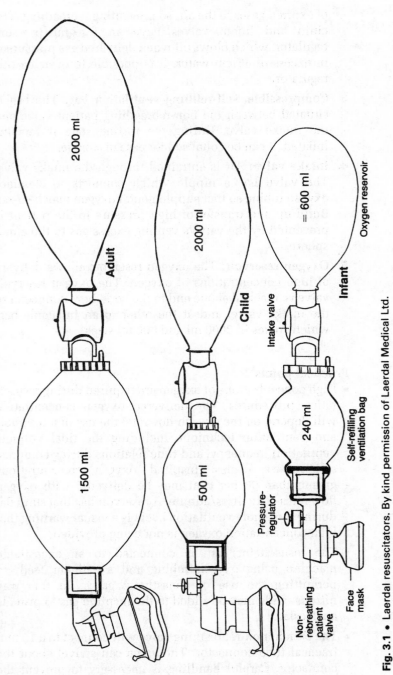

Fig. 3.1 • Laerdal resuscitators. By kind permission of Laerdal Medical Ltd.

of expired gases to the air, so preventing rebreathing. The child and infant valves have an integral pressure regulator, which blows off when delivered gas pressure is in excess of 45 cm water. It is possible to override this regulator.

3. **Compressible, self-refilling ventilation bag:** The bag is situated between the non-rebreathing patient valve and the intake valve. During the resting state it remains inflated. It can be collapsed for ease of storage.

4. **Intake valve:** Air is entrained through the intake valve. The valve has a nipple which connects to standard oxygen tubing so that supplemental oxygen may be used. Build-up and transfer of high pressure to the patient is prevented by the valve's venting excess gas to the atmosphere.

5. **Oxygen reservoir:** The oxygen reservoir allows delivery of high concentrations of oxygen. The oxygen reservoir valve is attached at one end to the wide-bore connector of the intake valve, and at the other to an inflatable bag, which comes in 2000 ml and 600 ml sizes.

Practical points
- High concentrations of oxygen are required during resuscitation procedures. The delivered oxygen concentration will depend on the oxygen flowrate, the use of a reservoir and ventilation technique including the tidal volume, ventilation frequency, and time relations during compression–release cycles. Inspired oxygen concentrations greater than 90 per cent may be delivered with oxygen flow rates of 10 litres/minute. A reservoir bag that stays flat during the whole ventilation cycle is a visual warning that high concentration oxygen is not being provided.

- The resuscitator can be connected to an anaesthetic machine using oxygen tubing and a catheter feed, so permitting the use of anaesthetic gases. In this way nitrous oxide may be added to the inspired gas to provide analgesia.

- The patient non-rebreathing valve will connect to a 15 mm tracheal tube connector. The valve can swivel about the connector. Careful handling is necessary to prevent the weight of the resuscitator pulling on the tracheal tube and dislodging it.

- Valves can stick, especially if cleaned with chemicals or autoclaved and not dried properly. With some designs parts of the valve can easily be removed and lost, so equipment must be checked carefully.

It is essential to be familiar with the characteristics of the self-inflating bags used in your hospital. Designs and safety features will vary, and a hospital is quite likely to have more than one make and model available. Some early models do not have oxygen reservoirs or pressure regulators on the paediatric non-rebreathing patient valve. With some designs the self-refilling bag will take a 15 mm connector, thus allowing the bag to be used without an expiratory valve. Always use a valve with a self-refilling bag.

Positive end expiratory pressure (PEEP) valves
These may be attached to the patient end of some makes of self-inflating bag. PEEP is most effectively applied if the patient is intubated. PEEP may be of value in patients suffering from heart failure, aspiration, thermal injury, or inhalation of irritant chemicals. PEEP can significantly reduce cardiac output.

Breathing systems
In the A & E department breathing systems are used during resuscitation procedures as well as for anaesthetizing patients. There are many different systems. Some are inappropriate for A & E use, and others should only be used by those with anaesthetic training. Classification of these systems is complicated. The diversity and complexity of the systems may lead to incorrect assembly, inconsistency with ordering new parts, and unfamiliarity with use (Table 3.3). This section will discuss some of the systems which A & E doctors are most likely to meet and may have to use in an emergency.

Table 3.3 • Characteristics of common anaesthetic breathing systems

System classification	Fresh gas flow needed to prevent rebreathing		Comment
	Spontaneous ventilation	Controlled ventilation	
Mapleson A (Magill or Lack)	80–90% of minute volume		Do not use for controlled ventilation
Mapleson D (Bain)	3 times minute volume	70 ml/kg/min with ventilation of 150 ml/kg/min	Only use for spontaneous breathing with capnography
Mapleson E & F (T-piece)	2.5–3.0 times minute volume (for child use 3 × (1000+100) ml/kg)	1000 + 100 ml/kg with ventilation of 1.5 times fresh gas flow	Minimum fresh gas flow 3 litres/min

Minute volume (adult) = 5000–6000 ml/min.

Basic components of a breathing system

All the systems have a source of oxygen, which may be from an anaesthetic machine, a wall supply, or the atmosphere. Carbon dioxide is eliminated by venting to the atmosphere or by using an absorber. A reservoir is used so that the system can accommodate the high peak flows during inspiration and expiration while using a low steady inflow of fresh gas. A reservoir requires a fresh gas flow. Except in the paediatric T-piece system a valve must always be present to prevent excessive circuit pressure and allow venting of exhaled gases. The system may include a source of anaesthetic gas and/or volatile anaesthetic.

Design of breathing systems (circuits)

There are two main groups of breathing systems. The first aims to provide minimal or no rebreathing by using high gas flows or a non-rebreathing valve. There is no provision for carbon dioxide absorption. They are sometimes known as semi-closed systems. The second group allows rebreathing. Carbon dioxide is removed by an absorber. Much lower gas flows can be used. These systems are sometimes known as closed, circle, or 'to and fro' systems. They should only be used by anaesthetists and they require in-line oxygen, carbon dioxide, and volatile agent monitoring. They should not be used for primary resuscitation.

Mapleson's classification of semi-closed breathing systems

The classification is based on the order in which the gas inlet, reservoir bag, anaesthetic tubing, valve, and face mask are assembled (Fig. 3.2). The Mapleson A or Magill attachment is commonly used for anaesthetizing spontaneously breathing patients. It may be present in resuscitation rooms, and A & E doctors should have a working knowledge of its structure, technique of use, and drawbacks. Mapleson C systems have been used for ventilation in primary resuscitation on general hospital wards. They are too complicated for use by minimally trained staff and should be replaced by a non-rebreathing manual resuscitator. The Lack and Bain coaxial systems are modifications of the Mapleson A and D systems respectively. They may be found in the A & E operating theatre but should only be used by those with anaesthetic training. The Mapleson E, T-piece system and its modifications are used in paediatric anaesthesia. A non-anaesthetist needing to ventilate a baby or child should use an appropriately sized manual non-rebreathing resuscitator with a pressure-limiting valve.

Mapleson A (Magill) system

The Mapleson A is the most efficient system for the spontaneously breathing patient, but carbon dioxide retention may occur with prolonged controlled ventilation. The dynamics can best be understood by considering three phases of ventilation: the inspiratory phase, the expiratory phase, and the expiratory pause.

Spontaneous ventilation
The circuit is initially full of fresh gas (Fig. 3.3(a)). As the patient breathes in, the gases are inhaled at a rate greater than the fresh gas flow. This causes partial emptying of the reservoir bag (Fig. 3.3(b)). During the first part of expiration the reservoir bag is partly empty, and the patient expires into the anaesthetic tubing, pushing the fresh gas in the tubing

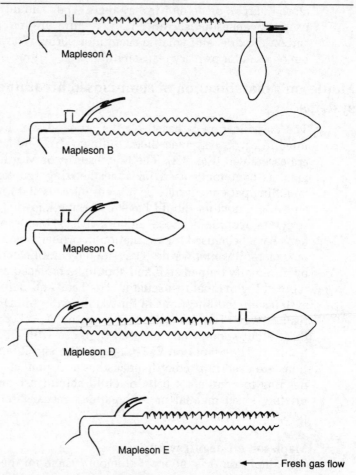

Fig. 3.2 ● Mapleson's classification of semi-closed breathing circuits.

back into the bag (Fig. 3.3(c)). The bag is refilled with fresh gas from the tubing and the anaesthetic machine before the exhaled gases can reach it. During the latter part of expiration the expired gases therefore leave through the expiratory valve, which now opens (Fig. 3.3(d)). During the expiratory pause the fresh gas flow forces more exhaled gas out through the expiratory valve. This phase is important to prevent rebreathing of exhaled alveolar gases. At the beginning of the next inspiration the patient will inhale a small amount of alveolar gas in the mask, followed by dead space gas and

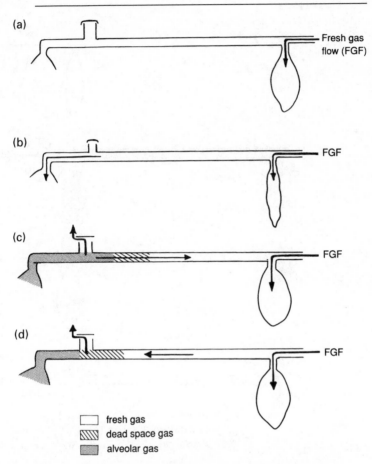

Fig. 3.3 • Mapleson A (Magill) system: spontaneous ventilation. (a) Circuit full of fresh gas; (b) inspiration and partial emptying of bag; (c) early expiration; and (d) late expiration.

then fresh gas. The fresh gas flow should be set at 80–90 per cent of the predicted minute volume, to prevent rebreathing.

Controlled ventilation
Different dynamics occur if the patient is manually ventilated using the Mapleson A system. The expiratory valve must be kept almost closed. During inspiration the bag is squeezed; fresh gases are directed into the patient, and some will escape through the expiratory valve (Fig. 3.4(a)).

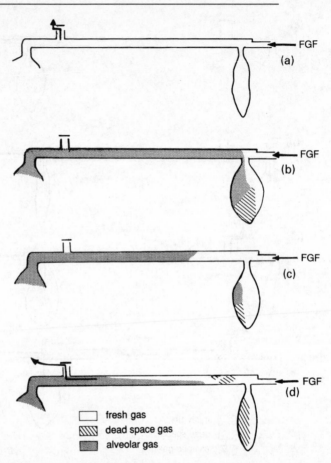

Fig. 3.4 • Mapleson A (Magill) system: controlled ventilation.
(a) Inspiration; (b) expiration; (c) subsequent early inspiration; and
(d) subsequent late inspiration.

Release of pressure on the bag initiates the start of expiration. At this stage the bag may be empty. The patient exhales up the anaesthetic tubing, but this time alveolar gas can reach the reservoir bag before the bag is filled with fresh gas from the tubing and the anaesthetic machine (Fig. 3.4*(b)*). There is a natural tendency to ignore the expiratory pause; thus the first gases to enter the patient on the next inspiration will be alveolar gases, followed by a mixture of fresh gas, dead space gas, and alveolar gas (Fig. 3.4*(c,d)*). Rebreathing therefore occurs with this system. It should not be used for controlled ventilation during primary resuscitation where a build-up of carbon dioxide may have serious consequences. For example, hypercarbia could exacerbate raised intra-cranial pressure in a head-injured patient. A self-inflating bag with a non-rebreathing valve should be used in these cases.

Lack coaxial system
This is the coaxial version of the Mapleson A system, which has the expiratory valve sited at the anaesthetic machine end of the system. The system has 1500 cm of 30 mm corrugated tubing and a 14 mm inner tube (Fig. 3.5). The outer tube supplies fresh gas to the patient from the reservoir bag, and the inner tube takes exhaled gas to be vented at the valve. The Lack system is suitable for spontaneous breathing, but not for controlled ventilation, since it behaves like a Mapleson A system.

Bain coaxial system
The system is a coaxial T-piece system designed like a Mapleson D system, with the expiratory valve and reservoir bag distal from the patient (Fig. 3.6). The system is 1800 cm of 22 mm diameter corrugated plastic tubing, through which runs a small-bore tube which delivers fresh gas to the patient. The patient's expired gases pass back through the outer tube to be vented at the valve. The Bain system is most efficient for controlled ventilation. A fresh gas flow of 70 ml/kg/min should be used to prevent rebreathing. The Bain system is not ideal for spontaneous breathing, and fresh gas flows from 150 ml/kg/min to three times the

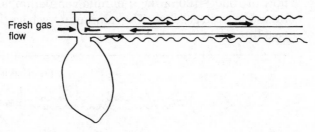

Fig. 3.5 • Lack coaxial system.

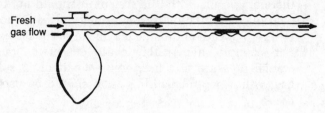

Fresh
gas flow

Fig. 3.6 • Bain coaxial system.

predicted minute volume have been advocated to prevent rebreathing.

Practical point
• The inner gas supply tube may become accidentally disconnected at the anaesthetic machine end of the system, causing a dangerous increase in dead space. The integrity of the inner tube must always be checked before using the Bain system.

Paediatric systems (Mapleson E and F)
Valveless T-piece systems are used for children under 20 kg. These have low resistance and low dead space, and are light. Spontaneous breathing is not commonly used in paediatric practice, except for brief anaesthesia. The addition of an open-ended 500 ml reservoir bag allows assisted or controlled ventilation using the T-piece system (Fig. 3.7). The performance of the system depends on the gas disposition at the T-piece junction. A fresh gas flow rate of 2.5–3.0 times the predicted minute volume is needed to prevent rebreathing during spontaneous breathing. During controlled ventilation normocapnia can be maintained by using a fresh gas flow of 1000 + 100 ml/kg if minute ventilation is at least 1.5 times the fresh gas flow. The minimum fresh gas flow should be 3 litres/min.

Fresh gas flow

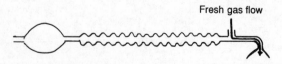

Fig. 3.7 • Paediatric T-piece.

Aids to airway maintenance and ventilation

These are used to supplement, not replace, basic airway management techniques. Any person using the equipment must be able to maintain an airway in an unconscious patient. This requires knowledge of positioning, the techniques of opening an airway, and the management of regurgitation or vomiting.

Oropharyngeal (Guedel) airways

These are made of disposable plastic and are available in different sizes (Table 3.4). There is a flange which lies in front of the lips and helps to keep the airway in place. The bite block is rigid, to prevent occlusion by the teeth. The curved, flattened tube holds the tongue clear of the posterior pharyngeal wall. Suction may be performed through the airway. Use of this airway is discussed on p. 141.

Nasopharyngeal airways

These are made of soft rubber or plastic. There is a flange which retains the tube at the nostril opening. Different makes have different sized flanges. A safety pin should be fixed through narrow flanges to prevent the airway slipping down the nostril. A curved tube with a bevelled end forms the communication with the nasopharynx. The airways come in various sizes, and are usually labelled in French gauge. Use of this airway is discussed on p. 143.

Table 3.4 • Oropharyngeal airways

Airway size	Patient
00	Baby
0	Infant
1	Child
2	Female
3	Male
4	Large adult

Face masks

Face masks similar to those used in anaesthesia have been designed for expired air ventilation. Various makes are available. The Laerdal pocket mask is a one-size transparent face mask with a mouthpiece. It folds away into a pocket-sized case. The mask is used when mouth to mouth ventilation is required. Its design prevents direct mouth contact with the patient, thus reducing the risk of infection. A one-way valve directs the patient's breath away from the rescuer. Supplemental oxygen may be given via oxygen tubing attached to an oxygen nipple. Mouth to mask ventilation is more efficient than poorly performed bag– mask–mouth ventilation. Use of a face mask is discussed on p. 169.

The laryngeal mask airway

The laryngeal mask airway (LMA) was first introduced into anaesthetic practice in 1988. It is now used for more than 40 per cent of elective anaesthetics in Britain. The LMA is a wide bore tube with an elliptical inflation cuff at the distal end which is designed to seal the hypopharynx close to the glottic opening (Fig. 3.8). In children, the LMA sits higher

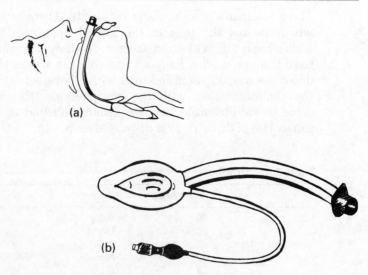

(a)

(b)

Fig. 3.8 • Laryngeal mask airway.

and may be more easily displaced than in adults. The LMA is available in paediatric and adult sizes (Table 3.5). There are standard and reinforced, flexible types. The LMA should be autoclaved after each use and each mask can be used about 40 times. The LMA provides a clear and secure airway leaving the operator's hands free. Its use does not require the same level of training and skill as tracheal intubation. However, placement is not always straightforward and requires practice. It is possible to position a LMA badly and obstruct the airway by folding the tip of the mask, rotating the mask, or displacing the epiglottis. A LMA does not protect the patient from aspiration of gastric contents or blood from facial trauma. However, evidence suggests that pulmonary aspiration during the use of a LMA is not common. It should not be used on unfasted patients unless the airway cannot be secured by other means. The LMA can be inserted when cricoid pressure is applied, but this makes placement more difficult. In normal patients ventilation is more effective and easier with a LMA than a bag and mask. Inflation pressure with a LMA should not exceed 20 cm water. Therefore the LMA is contraindicated in patients who require high inflation pressures to ventilate their lungs. The LMA has been used in patients with unstable necks, when access to the airway is limited or difficult. It has also been used in patients who are difficult to intubate, either as an alternative to tracheal intubation or as a guide for a bougie or fibre-optic laryngoscope. The LMA has been used by medical, nursing, and paramedical staff in the management of cardiopulmonary arrest. The LMA may be easier to use than a bag and mask and therefore less likely to lead to gastric insufflation and regurgitation. A multicentre study suggests that aspiration of gastric contents during the use of the LMA in resuscitation may not be a practical problem. Proper training

Table 3.5 • Sizes and cuff volumes for laryngeal mask airway

Size	Use	Cuff volume (ml)
1	Neonate/infant < 6.5 kg	2–4
2	Infant 6.5–15 kg	10
2.5	Child 15–30 kg	15
3	Child 30–35 kg/small adult	20
4	Adult	30
5	Large adult	40

in the use of the LMA and regular practice with it are needed if it is to be used in a resuscitation setting. Tracheal intubation is still the "gold standard" for ensuring ventilation and protecting the airway.

Tracheal tubes

Tracheal tubes may be cuffed or uncuffed. The cuff prevents gas leakage or aspiration around the tube, while also helping to hold it in place. The cuff is inflated using an air-filled syringe via a small-bore side tube. The cuff should be inflated until a leak is just prevented. This usually requires 5–10 ml air with the correct size of tube. Cuff inflation is indicated by a small inflatable 'pilot' balloon on the side tube. Escape of air from the cuff is prevented by a bung or a self-sealing valve at the end of the cuff tube. This opens when the syringe is inserted and closes with its removal. Cuffed tracheal tubes are used in adults in whom the narrowest part of the larynx is at the glottic opening. In children the cricoid cartilage is the narrowest portion and thus a cuffed tube is not needed. Noncuffed tubes should be used in children, since cuffed tubes could cause laryngeal and tracheal trauma. Plastic tubes come prepacked and must be cut to the appropriate length (Table 3.6). Tracheal tubes may be introduced via the oral or nasal route. The latter is less commonly used and requires a longer tube and added expertise at insertion. Plastic tracheal tubes are supplied with

Table 3.6 • Tracheal tube dimensions

Age	Internal diameter (mm)	Length (cm) Oral	Nasal
Premature neonate	2.5	11.0	14.0
0–4 weeks	3.0	11.0– 11.5	14.0– 14.5
1–6 months	3.5	11.5– 12.0	14.5– 15.0
0.5–1.0 year	4.0	12.0– 12.5	15.0– 15.5
1–2 years	4.5	12.5– 13.0	15.5– 16.0
2–4 years	5.0	13.0– 13.5	16.0– 16.5
4–5.5 years	5.5	13.5– 14.0	16.5– 17.0
5.5–7.5 years	6.0	14.5– 15.5	17.5– 18.5
7.5–9.0 years	6.5	15.5– 16.5	18.5– 19.5
> 9.0 years	7.0	15.6– 21.0	19.5– 24.0
Adult female	7.5– 8.5	21.0– 23.0	24.0– 26.0
Adult male	9.0– 10.0	23.0– 25.0	26.0– 28.0

standard 15 mm connectors which fit on to a standard resus-citator non-rebreathing valve or the appropriate catheter mount. Tracheal intubation is discussed on p. 146.

Practical points

• Always check the cuff before use. A tube with a damaged cuff must be replaced. Always ensure that the cuff is com-pletely deflated after checking for leaks. A partially inflated cuff can hinder intubation.

• Always check the tube has been cut to the correct length. Too short a tube may slip out of the trachea, risking hypoxaemia and aspiration. Too long a tube may result in bronchial intubation and hypoxaemia. Check the tube has been cut in the correct place. Tubes have been found cut at the patient rather than the connector end.

• Always check that the correct tracheal tube connector and catheter mount are available. These can get mixed up, making it difficult to connect the patient to an anaesthetic breathing system. Also ensure any suction portal is closed.

• Tracheal tubes must be carefully lubricated with sterile gel before use.

Laryngoscopes

A variety of laryngoscopes are available. Personal preference and hospital policy play a large part in what is used. During anaesthetic training it is useful to get experience with as many different types as possible. In the A & E department the types should be restricted to a minimum. It is essential that these should be interchangeable. A difficult emergency intubation is not the time to find that the large blade does not fit on any of the available handles.

The most commonly used adult laryngoscope is the Mac-intosh curved folding laryngoscope. This has four sizes of blade, large adult (no. 4), adult (no. 3), child (no. 2), and infant (no. 1). In practice there is little difference between the two smaller sizes, and once a child is about two years old an adult blade can often be used. The large adult blade is essential for occasional difficult intubations, and should always be available. The McCoy laryngoscope has an adjustable tip which may be useful for difficult intubations. Straight blades are sometimes preferred for difficult intubations and this is usually the blade of choice for children under six months. Blades may be attached by a screw (Longworth) fitting or a hook. The screw fitting is cumbersome if a rapid blade change is required. The hook fitting can be changed more easily, and is the fitting of choice for A & E use. Different types of blade will have different light carriers, which may not be interchangeable. The best laryngoscopes utilize a fibre-optic light source. Different bulbs may also be required. Use leak-proof batteries. Plastic laryngoscopes have fixed blades, with the light switch on the handle. This type is useful for pre-hospital care and 'MAJAX' packs.

Practical points

- Always check that the laryngoscope is working before use. In some situations reliance has to be put on a daily check of equipment, which may be overlooked. It is therefore mandatory to have a spare laryngoscope immediately available.

- A laryngoscope will not work if the batteries are flat, the bulb or light carrier becomes loosened from its connection, the spiral spring in the battery carrier is lost, or there is a loose connection within the unit.

Intubating stylets

These are fairly rigid and may be of copper or plastic-coated metal. They can be bent to the required shape. They help prevent tracheal tubes being distorted or deviated during insertion, and are particularly useful in difficult intubations. Different diameters are available.

Practical point

- Never allow the end of an intubating stylet to protrude past the level of the tracheal tube, as this may traumatize the airway.

Gum-elastic bougies

This is less rigid and longer than a stylet. It may be used as an aid during difficult intubation. It is introduced into the laryngeal opening, to serve as a guide for the tracheal tube, which is 'railroaded' over it. It is much less traumatic than a stylet, and can be introduced directly into the trachea.

Magill forceps

These are useful to help placement of a tracheal tube or naso-gastric tube under direct vision. They can also be used to remove foreign bodies from the mouth or pharynx under direct vision. Different sizes are available for adults and children.

Practical point
• Never hold the cuff of a tracheal tube in the forceps, since this may puncture the cuff.

Aids to difficult intubation

Intubation may be facilitated by transillumination techniques and cricothyroid puncture with catheter-guided intubation., These methods are only useful when the operator is experienced and have very little place in the A & E department. A fibre-optic laryngoscope may be used to enter the larynx and a tube may then be 'railroaded' over it. The use of fibre-optic instruments needs time and practice, and has only a small place in an emergency situation.

Suction

This is essential for airway maintenance. The three essential parts of a suction apparatus are the source of vacuum, the reservoir, and the delivery tubing. The efficiency of suction apparatus depends upon the degree of negative pressure produced and the diameter of the delivery tube. Suction may be provided by wall supply, electric motor, pressurized gas, foot pump, or hand pump. The latter is excellent for use in pre-hospital care or during patient transfer. A large catheter is most efficient for clearing profuse blood or vomit from the mouth. Finer catheters may be directed down airways or tracheal tubes. To reduce the risk of causing airway damage in children avoid using too large a catheter down the tracheal tube (Table 3.7).

Practical points
• Patient positioning, including elevating the foot of the trolley, may be required to supplement the use of suction.

Table 3.7 • Suction catheter sizes for tracheal tubes

Tracheal tube (internal diameter, mm)	Suction catheter (French gauge)
3.0	6.0
4.0	6.0
5.0	8.0
6.0	8.0
7.0	10.0
8.0	12.0
9.0	14.0
10.0	14.0

- Introduce suction catheters carefully. Rough use, particularly in small children, can produce laryngospasm and bleeding.
- Prolonged use of suction may cause airway collapse and hypoxaemia.
- Bradycardia may occur during tracheal suction.
- Always have more than one type of suction available in case of primary system failure. Hand powered suction is useful as back-up.

Oxygen masks

There are many different designs of oxygen mask. Inspired oxygen concentration may be controlled by the oxygen flow rate and mask design; but in some devices it will also be affected by the patient's inspiratory flow rate and expiratory pause. Some masks have a significant dead space. Masks designed around the Venturi principle can deliver a predictable oxygen concentration. The most commonly used face masks cannot deliver a concentration greater than 60 per cent. This is totally inadequate for the resuscitation of trauma patients, who require a concentration of greater than 85 per cent. Oxygen masks with a reservoir can deliver high oxygen concentrations.

Humidification

During long-term use inspired gases should be humidified. This is especially important in patients with chest problems, and it helps to maintain body temperature. Humidification does not have a routine place in A & E practice.

Maintenance of anaesthetic equipment

Anaesthetic machines, ventilators, and temperature compensated vaporizers should be serviced regularly by competent engineers. In addition the anaesthetist must carry out basic checks before using an anaesthetic machine. It is best to follow a set routine, so that nothing is forgotten.

Routine for checking anaesthetic apparatus

The use of checklists and associated procedures is an integral part of anaesthetic practice. The routine for checking anaesthetic apparatus set out by the Anaesthetists of Great Britain and Ireland in 1997 is widely accepted by the profession. It should be used in conjunction with preanaesthesia checking recommendations from manufacturers. To make it practically possible in every case, it should be able to be performed in a few minutes. It is mandatory that every anaesthetic machine has an oxygen analyser to prevent hypoxic mixtures being delivered and detect wrongly filled oxygen cylinders or reservoirs and incorrect pipeline connections. A written log should be attached to every machine so that a note of the checks performed can be made. The "first user check after engineering" is particularly important. Checking of anaesthetic apparatus, ventilators, breathing systems, and monitoring equipment is the responsibility of the anaesthetist and should not be delegated. An important part of checking is familiarization with any new equipment using instruction manuals. Before starting a case, the anaesthetist must ensure that they fully understand the equipment, especially if it is assembled in an unfamiliar way. The following is a suggested checklist.

1. Check that all equipment is plugged in to the mains supply and switched on.

2. Check that there is an oxygen analyser switched on, checked and calibrated. Monitor the output from the common gas outlet.

3. Check that the appropriate gas pipelines are connected and apply a "tug test". Check that there is an adequate supply of oxygen, including a reserve cylinder. Check that adequate supplies of other gases are available and connected properly. Turn all cylinders off. Carbon dioxide cylinders should not be connected routinely. Check that all pipelines pressure gauges register 400 kPa

4. Check that the flowmeters and the oxygen bypass control are working correctly. Use the oxygen analyser to confirm gas composition at the common gas outlet.

5. Check that the vaporizers are adequately filled and seated correctly. Check for leaks by temporary occlusion of the common gas outlet with the vaporizers on and off. Then turn the vaporizers off. If a vaporizer is changed at any stage these tests MUST be repeated.

6. Check the breathing system visually and secure all connections. Each breathing system has different potential problems and should be checked with these in mind. Occlude the patient port and compress the reservoir bag to pressure test the breathing system. Check the adjustable expiratory pressure-limiting valve. Ensure that unidirectional valves are working properly. If very low fresh gas flows in a circle system are planned, then the monitoring of oxygen concentration in the inspiratory limb, end-tidal carbon dioxide, and anaesthetic agent is mandatory.

7. Check the ventilator and set it for use. Make sure that the pressure relief valve and disconnection alarm are working. Always ensure that another means of ventilation is available (for example a self-inflating bag).

8. Check that the scavenging system is switched on and working.

9. Check that all ancillary equipment, including the suction machine, is working adequately. Make sure that the patient can rapidly be placed in a head down position.

10. Check all monitoring equipment and set the default alarms appropriately.

Safety during anaesthesia

Anaesthesia produces many possible hazards for patients and staff, including electric shock, fire or explosion, pollution of the environment with potentially harmful substances, and the possibility of infection with dangerous pathogens. Maintenance of standards of safe practice helps to reduce risks.

Electrical safety

If a voltage is applied between two contacts placed on the-body surface a current flows, the amount of which depends on the impedance of the pathway between the points, and which follows the path of lowest impedance. The resistance between the skin and the underlying tissue varies with local conditions, and may be mega-ohms ($m\Omega$) or kilo-ohms ($k\Omega$). Resistance is reduced in wet or broken skin and by the application of conductive jelly (when resistance may be as low as 300 Ω). The effect of an applied voltage depends on the current generated. At 0.5–2.0 mA tingling is discernible, at 15–100 mA muscle contraction occurs, and at 50 mA–2 A ventricular fibrillation develops. A higher current is needed to produce the same effect when direct rather than alternating current is applied. The effect of the current also depends upon its frequency. When very high frequency is used, as with diathermy, large currents pass through the body without adverse effects.

A live wire in a mains powered appliance carries the current as a single phase alternating supply at 50 Hz and 240 volts with respect to earth. A neutral wire carries the returning load current, and is nearly at earth potential. If an earth wire is present it should be at the local earth potential. The earth wire is there to provide a path for leakage currents arising from capacitive and inductive coupling between live and earthed parts of the appliance. The earth wire is normally connected to the metal case of the appliance, so that the case remains earthed if a live part of the equipment accidentally comes into contact with the case. Eventually, if the current becomes large enough, a fuse or circuit breaker operates, cutting off the flow of current.

Manufacturers of electromedical equipment are guided by regulations issued by the Department of Health and the British Standards Insitution. Leakage of electric current may lead to interference with monitoring equipment, fires and explosions in the presence of flammable substances, or electrocution. Accidental electric shock may arise through several different mechanisms, and may cause nerve damage, burns, or ventricular fibrillation. A current flows through a person who completes a circuit between a live and a neutral or a live and an earth wire. The current will be limited by the impedance of the pathway and the rating of any fuses. If a fault develops in equipment, a current may reach an anaesthetized patient through ECG electrodes or contact with any conducting material which forms part of the circuit. One of the commonest faults in equipment is the accidental disconnection of the earth wire, which goes unnoticed until another fault develops, causing the appliance's casing or some other accessible part to become live, giving the patient or a staff member an electric shock. Safety can be increased by isolating the electrical supply to the equipment from earth by using an isolating transformer.

If there is a direct connection between the environment and the patients' heart, such as a pacing wire, a Seldinger-wire, or a saline-filled central line, microelectrocution can occur with a relatively small current. Ventricular fibrillation may occur if 50 μA pass down a small electrode in contact with the ventricular wall. Small leakage currents of this order may arise when equipment is functioning normally. Great care must be taken when handling lines which lead directly into a patient's heart, and the possibility of microshock should be considered. If there are different appliances connected to the patient, each with a different earth, there is the potential for earth leakage currents even if the equipment is working normally. These are a possible source of microshock, and can be prevented by the use of isolation transformers.

Static electricity is a hazard if flammable anaesthetics are in use. As flammable anaesthetic agents are not needed in the A & E department, full antistatic precautions are now superfluous.

The following measures should be used routinely to promote electrical safety:

- Mains operated equipment must be effectively earthed and plugged into power sockets sharing a common earth.

- Battery operated equipment should not be earthed and should be insulated to prevent accidental earth connections.

- Equipment must be maintained to prevent accidental disconnection of the earth wire.

- The patient should be isolated from conductive material.

- Care must be taken not to touch electrical equipment or earthed metal objects when handling lines with a direct connection to the patient's heart.

- Areas where antistatic facilities are not provided should be clearly marked.

- Defibrillators should be used carefully, after proper training, as these are a potential source of electric shock to staff.

Fires and explosions

A fire or explosion needs three conditions to occur: a flammable agent, a gas which supports combustion (oxygen or nitrous oxide), and a source of ignition of greater than 1 μjoule (static electricity, monitoring apparatus, or a hot light source). Anaesthetic fires and explosions are much less common following the widespread acceptance of intravenous and non-flammable volatile anaesthetic agents as standard. There is no justification for the use of explosive anaesthetic agents such as ether in the A & E department. Care should be taken when flammable agents are used for other purposes, for example ether for skin cleaning or ethyl chloride for local anaesthesia. Glyceryl trinitrate patches must be removed before defibrillation, because of the potential for explosion.

Pollution and scavenging of waste gases

Many occupational health problems have been ascribed to breathing a polluted atmosphere. It is not known whether chronic exposure to low levels of anaesthetic agents is harmful. Nitrous oxide inactivates vitamin B12 and prevents it from facilitating the synthesis of folate, methionine, and thiamine. Nitrous oxide has been implicated as a cause of morbidity amongst dentists and anaesthetists. Toxicity can occur in dentists exposed to quite high nitrous oxide concentrations in unscavenged environments. Neuropathies are seen after prolonged occupational exposure or abuse of nitrous oxide. Occasional cases of anaesthetists with halothane hepatitis due to exposure at work have been reported. Higher rates of spontaneous abortion, low birth-weight babies, and a preponderance of female children have been reported in female theatre staff and the wives of male anaesthetists, but the relationship of these findings to pollution is not firmly established.

The regulations of control of substances hazardous to health (COSHH, 1989) address the issue of pollution in the working environment. Inhalational agents escaping from anaesthetic equipment or exhaled by a patient are a source of contamination. The level of pollution depends upon the anaesthetic technique used, gas flow, ventilation of the room, leaks in anaesthetic equipment, and the use of scavenging systems. The location of the measuring apparatus is important when assessing the exposure to inhalational agents. The area around the anaesthetist may have levels up to five times greater than those anticipated from calculations. The breathing zone of an anaesthetist in an unscavenged environment may have 100–5000 parts per million (ppm) nitrous oxide and 1–50 ppm halothane. In operating theatres with anaesthetic gas-scavenging systems (AGSSs) and recovery areas the concentrations are 10–100 ppm nitrous oxide and 0.2–3 ppm halothane. The COSHH regulations state minimum rates for air supply and weighted average exposure concentrations for volatile anaesthetics as

- nitrous oxide: 100 ppm
- isoflurane: 50 ppm
- enflurane: 20 ppm
- halothane: 10 ppm

Although a relationship between chronic exposure to anaesthetic agents and ill health is not confirmed, it is recommended that pollution is minimized. AGSSs should be used routinely and vaporizers must be filled and emptied using closed systems. Connections for AGSSs are 30 mm to prevent confusion with breathing systems. Passive AGGSs allow waste gases to be conveyed to the outside atmosphere by low resistance tubing. Active AGSSs are used more commonly and utilize negative pressure to remove wastes. AGGSs have a collecting system which delivers gases from breathing circuits or ventilator outlets to a transfer system. Collection attachments for paediatric circuits allow spillage into transfer tubing. The tranfer system must have a positive pressure release valve to prevent high pressure being delivered back to the patient or ventilator. The waste gases then pass to a receiving system with a reservoir which has positive and negative pressure release valves. A bacterial filter is incorporated in the system to prevent infection. A disposal system carries gases from the receiving system to the outside atmosphere.

Infection control in anaesthesia

Single-use items are being used increasingly in anaesthetic practice. These include tracheal tubes, airways, breathing systems, reservoir bags, and soda-lime canisters. Ventilators and non-disposable breathing systems may be protected by low resistance bacterial and viral filters. Breathing systems can be a reservoir for organisms, especially if moisture is present. A sterile breathing system should be used for each patient. Cleaning guidelines may vary between hospitals. It is best to take advice from the hospital infection control officer or contact the manufacturer. Handwashing is the single most important infection control measure.

Further reading

Association of Anaesthetists of Great Britain and Ireland (1975). Advice to members from the Council: pollution of the atmosphere in operating theatres. *Anaesthesia*, **30**, 697– 9.

Association of Anaesthetists of Great Britain and Ireland (1997). *Checklist for anaesthetic apparatus 2*. A A G B I, London.

European Resuscitation Council (ERC) (1996). *Resuscitation*, **31**,201–30.

Halsey, M. J. (1991). Occupational health and pollution from anaesthetics:a report of a seminar. *Anaesthesia*, **46**, 486–8.

Hull, C. J. (1978). Electrocution hazards in the operating theatre. *British Journal of Anaesthesia*, **50**, 647– 57.

Moyle, J. T. B. (1990). Electrical safety. *Anaesthesia Reviews* **7**, (ed.K. Kaufman). Churchill Livingstone, Edinburgh.

Multicentre Trial (coordinated by P. J. F. Basket) (1994). The use of the laryngeal mask airway by nurses during cardiopulmonary resuscitation. *Anaesthesia*, **49**, 3–7.

Parbrook, G. D., Davis, P. D., and Parbrook, E. O. (1990). *Basic physics and measurement in anaesthesia*, (4th edn.). Butterworth-Heinemann, Oxford.

Redfern, N. (1990). Morbidity amongst anaesthetists. *British Journal of Hospital Medicine*, **43**, 377– 81.

Vickers, M. D. (1978). Fire and explosion hazards in operating theatres. *British Journal of Anaesthesia*, **50**, 659– 64.

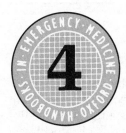

CHAPTER 4

Infection risks during anaesthesia

Key points in infection risks during anaesthesia

- Assume that all patients are potential carriers of communicable diseases.

- Adopt precautions to prevent transmission of infection including goggles, gloves, fluid-impervious gowns, and masks. Avoid injuries by careful handling of needles and blades and the use of biohazard containers.

- All staff who may come into contact with blood or body fluids should be immunized against hepatitis B. If a non-immune person is contaminated he or she must be treated with immunoglobin followed by active immunization.

- Counselling may be needed for professionals who are at risk of contracting a communicable disease, for example after a needle-stick injury.

There is a risk of contracting infectious diseases during anaesthesia, especially in a trauma situation. Routine hygiene and sterilization are adequate protection against the transmission of tuberculosis. However, consideration must be given to the increased incidence of multiresistant tuberculosis. More serious infections include hepatitis B and human immunodeficiency virus (HIV). However, other more occult infections are also a problem, for example hepatitis C and D. As it is impossible to predict which patients may be infected, universal precautions should be adopted in all cases.

Hepatitis B

Hepatitis B is very infectious, and can be transmitted by blood or sexual contact. The infection can be carried by small quantities of blood, which may be present in body fluids such as saliva. Transmission of infection in health care workers often occurs through the skin as a result of needle-stick injuries or via small abrasions. The risk of seroconversion after occupational exposure is 5–30 per cent. Exposure to hepatitis B and seroconversion may be asymptomatic. The incubation period is prolonged, and acute hepatitis, chronic active hepatitis, cirrhosis, or hepatoma may develop after infection. Five to ten per cent of those infected become carriers of the virus and have hepatitis surface antigen in the blood. There are 200 million carriers of hepatitis B in the world. There are about 2000 new cases each year in Britain; 1 in 500 of the adult population in the UK are carriers. It is especially prevalent in intravenous drug abusers, prostitutes, homosexuals, prisoners, inmates of long term institutions, and patients who have had multiple blood product transfusions. The level of infectivity can be determined serologically; the presence of hepatitis B surface antigen e is associated with high infectivity. Safe and effective vaccines are available to protect against hepatitis B, and all staff who come into contact with blood or body fluids must be immunized. If a non-vaccinated person becomes contaminated with infected blood they must be given a dose of hepatitis B immunoglobulin as rapidly as possible, and this should be repeated 30 days later. They should simultaneously receive active immunization with hepatitis B vaccine. The response to vaccination must be checked serologically.

AIDS

The highest incidence of HIV infection is amongst homosexual men and intravenous drug abusers. Heterosexual transmission of the disease is becoming an important mode of infection. At present AIDS is an incurable disease with no possibility of vaccination to prevent infection. In 1992 there were about 50,000 HIV-positive people in Britain. HIV has been isolated in body fluids such as saliva, blood, tears, urine, cerebrospinal fluid, semen, synovial fluid, and breast milk. Transmission usually occurs sexually, transplacentally, or via infected blood. Infection from saliva has not been reported. Although HIV is less easily transmitted than hepatitis B, health-care workers have been infected by needle-stick injuries. The risk of seroconversion after occupational exposure is 0.39 per cent. There is some research suggesting that prophylactic administration of zidovudine given quickly after exposure to HIV virus may be helpful. It should be recognized that any patient may present an infection risk and precautions to minimize the risk of transmission should be routine.

Precautions against transmission of infection

The following guidelines should be observed when dealing with infected patients, and many of them can be applied routinely to decrease the overall risk of cross-infection.

- Needles and other 'sharps' must be placed in a suitable container, to be burned later. 'Sharps' must never be handed from person to person, but should be placed in a tray. Needles must never be resheathed, as this is the commonest cause of needle-stick injury.
- Proper biohazard bins must be used for all 'sharps'.
- If a needle-stick injury occurs or an abrasion becomes contaminated with blood, bleeding should be encouraged, and the skin should be washed thoroughly with soap and water. The injury must not be sucked.
- Any cuts or abrasions on the skin should be covered with waterproof dressings, as they are a potential site for the entry of infection. If there are large areas of abrasion or dermatitis, gloves should be worn.
- Gloves, a plastic apron, mask, and eye protection should be worn.
- As the hepatitis virus and HIV are not airborne the parts of the breathing system outside the patient do not constitute

an infection risk to the staff and anaesthetist. All breathing systems should be routinely protected with a bacterial filter. The pleated type with hydrophobic membrane are the only suitable filters. The filter must be changed between patients.

- As much equipment as possible should be disposable. Any equipment which is autoclavable should be sterilized in this way. Other equipment should be sterilized with freshly prepared glutaraldehyde, washed in soap and water, and then left to soak in glutaraldehyde for 3 hours. Contaminated floors and surfaces should be washed with a fresh solution of 1 per cent hypochlorite.

- Disposable material from an infected patient should be placed in red bags and sent immediately for incineration.

- The number of staff and the amount of equipment in the room should be kept to a minimum when dealing with infected cases.

- If a member of staff is contaminated with potentially infected material, they should immediately contact the occupational health department. Blood sampling, administration of vaccines, and other medication should then be arranged. Longer term follow-up and counselling for staff may be needed.

Care should be taken to avoid the risk of cross-infection when dealing with all patients, and not just those who are known to be infected, or at high risk of being infected, with dangerous pathogens. Known infected patients should probably be anaesthetized for elective procedures in the main operating theatres rather than in the A & E department. It is then easier to put the patient last on the operating list, clean and rest the theatre afterwards, and allow staff to dispose of protective clothing. The A & E department should be set up to deal with potentially infectious patients during an emergency situation. The same routine for cleaning and sterilizing equipment which is used in the operating theatres must be applied in the A & E setting.

Further reading

Association of Anaesthetists of Great Britain and Ireland (1988). *AIDS and hepatitis B. Guidelines for Anaesthetists.* A A G B I, London.

Association of Anaesthetists of Great Britain and Ireland (1992). *HIV and other blood borne viruses – a guide for the anaesthetist,* A A G B I, London.

Lee, K. G. and Soni, N. (1986). AIDS and anaesthesia. *Anaesthesia,* **41**, 1011–16.

Meredith, S., Watson, J. M., Citron, K. M., Cockcroft, A. and Darbyshire, J. H. (1996). Are health care workers in England and Wales at increased risk of tuberculosis? *British Medical Journal,* **313**, 522–5.

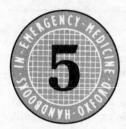

CHAPTER 5

Assessment of patients, general anaesthesia, and monitoring during anaesthesia

Key points in assessment, general anaesthesia and monitoring

- A & E staff should assess each patient before contacting the anaesthetist: checklists can be useful.
- Anaesthetists should only give anaesthetics in the A & E department if they are happy about the condition of the patient and the equipment and assistance available.
- Rapid sequence induction is mandatory in patients who may have a full stomach or intra-abdominal pathology. It is also advisable in obese patients and in those given opioid analgesics.
- Monitoring apparatus should be checked before use.

Assessment for general anaesthesia

Careful preoperative assessment of the patient is an essential prerequisite for safe anaesthesia of both urgent and elective cases. Much time can be saved if the staff of the A & E department thoroughly evaluate the general health and specific problems of each patient before contacting the anaesthetist, perhaps by using checklists (Table 5.1). Any appropriate investigations should be performed. The anaesthetist may be able to make recommendations over the telephone to improve the condition of the patient before making a more formal assessment. Good communication between the anaesthetist and the A & E staff is fundamental to safe and efficient anaesthesia.

No patient should receive elective anaesthesia without prior discussion with their anaesthetist. A preoperative anaesthetic assessment allows the mutual transfer of useful information, permits the patient to form a relationship with the anaesthetist, and allows patients the opportunity to ask questions. The reduction in anxiety produced by a sympathetic visit from the anaesthetist often renders premedication unnecessary.

Fitness for general anaesthesia

The American Society of Anesthesiologists (ASA) has defined a system of classification of the preoperative state of patients which has been widely adopted (Table 5.2). This was not designed for risk assessment, but the chance of a patient having a problem during general anaesthesia correlates well with ASA status. Patients for elective general anaesthesia in the A & E Department should be ASA I or II.

Table 5.1 • Checklist for preoperative assessment of patients in A & E

Patient details		Medical history	
Age		Cardiac disease	YES/NO
Weight		Respiratory disease	YES/NO
Time of last drink		Airway problem	YES/NO
Time of last food		GI problem	YES/NO
Drugs		Other illness	YES/NO
Allergies		Details	
Blood pressure			
Smoker	YES/NO		
Dentures/crowns/loose teeth			

Anaesthetic history		Present problem	
Previous GA	YES/NO	Trauma	YES/NO
Problems		Drugs given in A & E	
Family GA history	YES/NO	Pregnant	YES/NO
Problems			

Table 5.2 • American Anesthesiologists Society classification of preoperative status

I	Healthy patient with no systemic diseases
II	A patient with a mild to moderate systemic disease process caused either by the condition to be treated surgically or other pathological process and which does not limit the patient's activity in any way, for example mild diabetic, treated hypertensive, heavy smoker
III	A patient with severe systemic disturbance from any cause which imposes a definite functional limitation on activity, for example ischaemic heart disease with a limited exercise tolerance, severe chronic obstructive airways disease
IV	A patient with severe systemic disease which is a constant threat to life, for example severe chronic bronchitis, advanced liver disease
V	A moribund patient who is unlikely to survive 24 hours with or without treatment

* E added to signify an emergency operation

History and examination

During preoperative assessment the cardiorespiratory systems must be evaluated for evidence of acute or chronic problems. A note of cigarette smoking should be made, as this increases airway irritability and reduces mucociliary clearance. The adequacy of mouth opening, dentition and the patency of the upper airway must be assessed carefully. There have been various methods used to predict difficult intubation. The Mallampti classification is based on examination of the oropharynx with the patient sitting upright opposite the assessor with the mouth fully open and tongue protruded. Laryngoscopy is likely to be difficult when viewing of the faucial pillars, uvula, and soft palate is obscured by the tongue. There are several scoring systems which try to predict difficulty with intubation, but most give a high proportion of false positive predictions. Since it is not possible to forsee difficult intubation reliably, emphasis should be on proficient use of a failed intubation drill. Cormack and Lehane classified four grades of intubation according to the view at laryngoscopy:-

- Grade 1: most of the glottis visible
- Grade 2: only the posterior aspect of the glottis visible
- Grade 3:no part of the glottis visible
- Grade 4:not even epiglottis visible.

Grades 3 and 4 pose possible difficulty with intubation. Symptoms and signs of haematological, renal, liver, neuro-muscular, metabolic, or endocrine disease should be noted. All women of childbearing age should be asked about the possibility of pregnancy and tested if necessary. Significant past medical history should be recorded. Patients should be weighed if possible. Examination must include assessment of the heart rate and rhythm, measurement of blood pressure, and careful chest ausculation. Psychological and social factors should be considered prior to giving general anaesthesia in the A & E Department.

Drug history

A careful drug history is mandatory. Drugs for the control of systemic illness, such as hypertension, epilepsy, or chest problems, should be taken prior to anaesthesia. Medication should not be omitted because a patient is fasting prior to anaesthesia. It is particularly important that patients receive preoperative doses of steroids and bronchodilators. The only agents which must not be taken prior to anaesthesia are oral hypoglycaemics, insulin, and monoamine oxidase inhibitors. Careful note should be made of known drug allergies.

Anaesthetic and family history

A history of a previous adverse reaction to local or general anaesthesia should be explored carefully. Difficulty with intubation, emesis, awareness, drug allergy, and slow re-covery are especially relevant. Prolonged apnoea, jaundice, or admission to an intensive care unit after anaesthesia is very significant, and justify deferring elective anaesthesia pending further information. Previous anaesthesia in members of the patient's family should be considered when conditions such as suxamethonium sensitivity and malignant hyperthermia may be discovered.

Investigations

Seventy-five per cent of ASA I and II patients do not need routine tests prior to anaesthesia. Unexpected abnormalities will be found in 10–11 per cent of patients but these will only alter management in 0.6 per cent of cases. Haemoglobin should be measured in patients with clinical evidence of bleeding or anaemia, menstruating women, and patients over 55 years. All Afro-Caribbean, Mediterranean, and Asian patients should have a sickle cell test. If the test is positive, elective anaesthesia must be deferred pending full electro-phoresis to differentiate sickle cell trait and disease. Urea and electrolytes should be measured in patients over 55 years, those with diabetes, those on cardiac drugs or diur-etics or when dehydration may be present. Blood glucose should be measured in diabetics and patients on steroids. All patients should have urinalysis. A pregnancy test may be needed. In 1979 the Royal College of Radiologists recom-mended that routine chest X-ray is unnecessary prior to anaesthesia. It may be desirable in certain situations, includ-ing acute respiratory distress, where metastatic disease is suspected, in chronic airways disease where no chest X-ray has been performed in the previous year, and where the possibility of tuberculosis exists. A preoperative chest X-ray influences the management of less than 1 per cent of ASA I and II patients. An ECG is only required if clinically indicated, for example in symptomatic patients, in those over the age of 50 years, and in diabetics over 40 years. Blood should be cross-matched if the patient has been bleeding or may require surgery involving a significant risk of blood loss. Clotting studies should be performed if clinically indicated.

Preparation for general anaesthesia

- Consent should be obtained for the anaesthetic and the procedure from the patient or his or her guardian.
- The patient should be dressed in a suitable gown to permit access to the chest and operative site. A wristband listing the patient's name, unit number, and any allergies should be applied.
- False teeth, dental plates, hearing aids, prostheses, contact lenses, jewellery, and nail polish should be removed.
- The patient should have nothing to eat or drink for 6 hours prior to anaesthesia. The reasons for this should be clearly explained to the patient. Patients with acid reflux or a

history of a hiatus hernia should receive antacid prophylaxis (ranitidine 300 mg orally or 50 mg intravenously 2 hours before anaesthesia, if time permits, and 30 ml 0.3 M sodium citrate 30 minutes before anaesthesia). Patients who ate or drank shortly before sustaining trauma or who have received opioids are especially at risk. The risk of aspiration of gastric contents is increased five-fold in emergency surgery compared to elective procedures in all age groups.

- Patients in pain should receive appropriate analgesia. Those waiting for anaesthesia should not be denied analgesic drugs, but their medication should be discussed with the anaesthetist.

- Patients who are nauseated or vomiting before anaesthesia should be given an appropriate antiemetic (see p. 251). Metoclopramide may be used to try to increase gastric emptying, but it cannot guarantee an empty stomach, and is particularly unreliable if opioids or atropine have been given.

- Patients who require antibiotic prophylaxis because of a history of rheumatic fever, heart defects, or prosthetic valves will be given these by the anaesthetist immediately before anaesthesia.

- Patients on long term steroids will sometimes need additional steroids, to be given by the anaesthetist immediately before anaesthesia.

- Patients who require prophylaxis against deep venous thrombosis will need to be admitted to hospital for their surgery.

Contraindications to elective anaesthesia in the A & E department

Cardiovascular problems
- Uncontrolled hypertension with a diastolic blood pressure of more than 100 mm Hg
- Ischaemic heart disease, especially with myocardial infarction within 3 months or unstable angina
- Valvular heart disease
- Heart failure which increases the risk of anaesthesia by up to 30-fold

- Congenital cardiac problems
- Circulatory shock
- Cerebrovascular disease
- Intracerebral aneurism

Respiratory problems
- Upper or lower respiratory tract infection
- Chronic obstructive airways disease
- Asthma
- Pneumothorax

Airway problems
- Predicted difficult intubation
- Dental abscess
- Cervical instability
- Airway obstruction
- Bleeding into the airway

Haematological problems
- Anaemia
- Sickle cell disease
- Clotting disorders or patients on anticoagulants

Renal or hepatic disease
- Renal failure
- Liver failure
- Electrolyte or metabolic derangement

Neuromuscular problems
- Myopathies, myasthenia, or myotonia
- Neurological diseases affecting airway competence and muscle power
- Raised intracranial pressure

Endocrine or metabolic problems
- Obesity with a body mass index (weight in kg/height in m^2) of 30 or more

- Poorly controlled diabetes mellitus
- Uncorrected hypothyroid or hypoadrenal states
- Uncontrolled hyperthyroidism
- Cachexia

Miscellaneous
- Pregnant patients
- Patients with recent burns or major muscle damage
- Patients who may transmit infections such as hepatitis B or HIV
- Psycho-social problems may preclude safe day-case anaesthesia
- Suxamethonium sensitivity
- Susceptibility to malignant hyperthermia

Premedication

Adults should not usually receive sedative premedication, as this may delay recovery. Patients in pain or with emetic problems should be given appropriate treatment before anaesthesia. They may need admission to hospital post-operatively. Premedication may be useful in children who become distressed whilst waiting for general or local anaesthesia. Oral midazolam 0.5–0.75 mg/kg may be useful, it can be mixed with paracetomol syrup (10mg/kg) for patients in pain. Parenteral premedication is not usually appropriate for paediatric patients. Application of local anaesthetic cream to the proposed sites of venepuncture or injection one hour before anaesthesia is important in preventing pain and distress.

Conclusion

The A & E department is a difficult environment for the trainee anaesthetist, because it is often isolated from the main areas where anaesthesia is given and where senior help is available. Trainee anaesthetists should only give anaesthesia in the A & E setting when they are totally happy with the condition of the patient and with the equipment and assistance available. If there is any doubt about the fitness of a patient for general anaesthesia, the decision should be made at a senior level, and a senior anaesthetist should then be present to supervise.

General anaesthesia for elective and emergency procedures

Elective cases

Elective general anaesthesia may be required in the A & E department. The patient may refuse to have local anaesthesia or be too young to cooperate. The patient's pathology or the presence of infection may make general anaesthesia more appropriate.

Before administering general anaesthesia it is important to check that the appropriate drugs are available and that the anaesthetic, monitoring, and resuscitation equipment is working. Suitably trained operating department practitioners should be present to help the anaesthetist, who should know where to reach senior help if it is required. The patient's identity, presenting problem and consent should be verified. A full history and examination must be performed on every patient who is to have a general anaesthetic (see p. 74). It is important to verify that the patient is fasted and to perform a final check of the dentition and the airway. Ensure that the patient has transport home. The patient and any carer present, must understand any instructions for postoperative care. If the patient is a child the parent should be encouraged to accompany the child during the induction of anaesthesia. However, if the parent is obviously not happy to do so, they must not be coerced.

Anaesthesia for elective procedures in the A & E department should be as simple as possible. Premedication should usually be avoided, as it may delay recovery. Analgesia may be needed if the patient has to wait for anaesthesia. Intravenous induction of anaesthesia is preferable to gaseous induction, as it is rapid and pleasant. If local anaesthetic cream is used most children will tolerate intravenous induction, but gaseous induction may be offered as an alternative. Propofol is the agent of choice, as it produces quick and complete recovery and does not have active metabolites. If possible, the use of muscle relaxants and intubation should be avoided in patients who are to be discharged home. Anaesthesia involving spontaneous breathing of oxygen, nitrous oxide, and a volatile anaesthetic agent from a mask and airway or a laryngeal mask is preferable. Sevoflurane and desflurane produce the most rapid recovery. Supplementation with non-steroidal antiinflammatory drugs or local anaesthetic blocks may be used to provide postoperative pain relief. Minimum monitoring standards must be adhered to during even a brief anaesthetic. Once the procedure is over the patient should be placed in the recovery position and supervised by trained staff until recovery is complete. The anaesthetist should remain with the patient until consciousness and complete control of the airway return.

Emergency cases

Sometimes anaesthesia and intubation are needed in an emergency situation in the A & E department, for example to maintain and protect the airway and provide adequate ventilation following head injury, burns or multiple trauma. The patient may have a full stomach, and is at risk of aspiration of gastric contents into the lungs. The priority is to secure the airway as rapidly and safely as possible whilst maintaining oxygenation. The only way to protect the airway is to intubate the patient with a cuffed tracheal tube (uncuffed in the case of a small child), which usually requires anaesthesia and muscle paralysis. Deeply unconscious patients may be intubated without anaesthesia and paralysis. If a patient has a gag reflex it is not possible to intubate smoothly without anaesthesia and paralysis. Attempts to intubate such a patient may result in regurgitation. It is dangerous to try to intubate a head injured patient without anaesthesia, because this produces a massive rise in intracranial pressure. In trauma the risk of cervical spine injury should always be considered. Those with multiple trauma, victims of high speed accidents, unconscious patients or those with blunt injury above the clavicle should have spinal immobilization. The need for total spinal immobilization should be remembered. Immobilization at the cervical spine increases the difficulty of tracheal intubation. Adequate oxygenation must be maintained in this situation.

Rapid sequence induction of anaesthesia

1. Check all drugs and equipment and have suction, laryngoscope, and tracheal tubes within easy reach.

2. Ensure that the assistants understand the principles of rapid sequence induction and spinal immobilization.

3. Explain the procedure to the patient.

4. Site an intravenous cannula.

5. Preoxygenate the patient by supplying 100 per cent oxygen via a mask with a tight seal. The time taken to denitrogenate the lungs totally is 7 minutes. The process is 80 per cent complete if 100 per cent oxygen is breathed at normal tidal volumes for 1 minute, this allows 3 minutes of apnoea in a normal person. Continuing preoxygenation for 3 minutes or taking a few vital capacity breaths almost doubles apnoea time to 5 minutes.

6. Give a dose of induction agent, usually thiopentone, which is predetermined from the patient's weight and general condition. Give the complete dose quickly, not titrated against effect, with the aim of producing rapid unconsciousness.

7. As the induction agent is being given ask the assistant to apply cricoid pressure. This is achieved by pressing firmly backwards on the ring of the cricoid cartilage to occlude the oesophagus. The assistant may use his or her other hand to support the back of the patient's neck. The use of cricoid pressure (Sellick's manœuvre) reduces the risk of regurgitation of stomach contents. The assistant must know that cricoid pressure must never be released until the anaesthetist states that it is safe to do so. If the patient begins to vomit actively the anaesthetist must instruct that cricoid pressure should be released, as oesophageal rupture may occur.

8. Give a generous dose of suxamethonium (100 mg in an adult) immediately after the induction agent, without waiting to observe the effect of the induction agent.

9. Keep the face mask tightly applied whilst the relaxant is working, and wait for paralysis to be complete. Do not manually ventilate the lungs, as this may inflate the stomach and increase the risk of regurgitation.

10. Intubate the patient and inflate the tracheal tube cuff as swiftly as possible. When the tube position is certain and the cuff is inflated allow the cricoid pressure to be released. If intubation is not possible follow the failed intubation drill (page 107).

Rapid sequence induction is mandatory if the patient may have a full stomach, in the presence of intra-abdominal pathology, or in patients with visceral pain, such as testicular torsion. It is advisable in obesity, or with a history of recent alcohol or opioid intake. Most children seem to arrive in the A & E department with full stomachs, therefore rapid sequence induction may be advisable for them.

Anaesthesia for cardioversion

Anaesthesia is required for cardioversion of conscious patients, and it should be performed by an anaesthetist. Single-handed sedation and cardioversion is hazardous, and only justified in an emergency. The appropriate anaesthetic technique is determined by the general health of the patient, the condition of the circulation, and whether or not the patient has a full stomach. A patient having planned cardioversion will usually have fasted and have a reasonable cardiac output. However, a patient requiring emergency cardioversion may have an unstable low cardiac output and be at risk of vomiting and aspiration. The need for cardioversion implies an underlying cardiac problem, and perhaps a fixed cardiac output. Induction of anaesthesia is slow in patients with a low cardiac output.

Inexperienced doctors may be tempted to give too much induction agent, in their anxiety to get the patient asleep quickly, and cause prolonged coma, drowsiness, or apnoea. Anaesthesia should be induced using a drug which preserves cardiovascular stability – the best agent probably being etomidate. Diazemuls or midazolam produce sedation slowly and leave the patient drowsy for much longer than etomidate.

Benzodiazepines are sometimes used by non-anaesthetists in urgent situations, but may cause hypotension and apnoea. If a patient with a full stomach requires urgent cardioversion one should use a rapid sequence induction technique using etomidate and suxamethonium. If there is any risk of regurgitation during cardioversion the airway must be protected by tracheal intubation. Adequate oxygenation is vital during anaesthesia for cardioversion, as hypoxia reduces the effectiveness of the procedure. Pulse oximetry should be used to ensure that oxygenation is optimal before the shock is delivered. Reliable venous access is required, since the infusion is liable to be dislodged during the procedure. Patients must be carefully monitored during the recovery period.

Monitoring during anaesthesia and recovery

Monitoring involves frequent observation of parameters to detect abnormalities or trends towards the abnormal. High standards of monitoring must be applied rigorously in all areas where anaesthesia is administered, including A & E departments. The most important safety feature is the presence of a suitably trained anaesthetist and assistant throughout. The use of monitoring equipment should not detract from the need for careful clinical observation.The anaesthetist must be familiar with the monitors. These should be checked and calibrated and have their alarms functional and their sensors sited appropriately prior to anaesthesia. Patients should be monitored during induction of anaesthesia, maintenance and recovery. Patients undergoing procedures under sedation also require monitoring. Monitoring is also important during transport of ill or unconscious patients. Undesirable trends should be treated promptly, and the anaesthetist should have a plan in the event of equipment failure.

Patient monitoring

Cardiovascular monitoring
All patients must have continuous ECG monitoring and intermittent recording of blood pressure during anaesthesia and recovery.

Capnography

Capnography uses infrared absorption to measure the concentration of carbon dioxide in gas mixtures aspirated from breathing systems by a simple tube attachment. End tidal carbon dioxide concentration provides an index of the arterial carbon dioxide concentration, and hence of the adequacy of alveolar ventilation. The carbon dioxide concentration should be measured as near to the airway as possible. A system which displays a trace, rather than a digital value, is preferable, as inaccuracies in sampling will be more obvious. Capnography gives an indication of oesophageal intubation, hyperventilation, disconnection, hypotension, air embolism (when the carbon dioxide concentration falls), and inadequate ventilation and malignant hyperthermia (when the carbon dioxide concentration rises). Portable carbon dioxide monitors are useful for intra- and interhospital transfer of patients. They should be small, robust, give an audible signal with each breath and have a good battery life.

Oximetry

Pulse oximetry is used to measure and display transcutaneous oxygen saturation from probes which clip on to fingers, toes, or ear lobes. Oximeters use light-emitting diodes and a photoabsorber to measure light absorption at two bandwidths. The technique depends on the difference in absorption between oxygenated and reduced haemoglobin, and is independent of haemoglobin concentration or skin pigmentation. Pulse oximeters have rapid response times, and are accurate to 1 per cent when the oxygen saturation is greater than 80 per cent. The accuracy may be compromised by dysfunctional haemoglobin such as carboxy or methaemoglobin, hyperbilirubinaemia, tricuspid incompetence, diagnostic dyes, and methaemoglobinaemia, when the saturation reads high. In low cardiac output states or vasoconstriction the oximeter may fail to pick up a signal. Intense light and patient movement may also lead to artefacts in monitoring. A fall in oxygen saturation is a late indication of problems, especially when the patient has been preoxygenated.

Neuromuscular monitoring

If a patient is given a muscle relaxant it is important to moniter this using a peripheral nerve stimulator. Clinical assessment of neuromuscular recovery, for example by grip strength or head lift, can be unreliable. A nerve stimulator applies a supramaximal stimulus to a peripheral nerve (such as the ulnar, facial, or common peroneal nerve) and the response may then be assessed visually, mechanically, or electrically. A train of four (TOF) supramaximal stimuli given at an interval of 0.5 seconds over a period of 2 seconds to assess the degree of block. The amplitude of the fourth response in relation to the first gives the TOF ratio. During a partial depolarizing block all four twitch heights will be of equal size. During a non-depolarizing block the TOF ratio begins to decrease when 75 per cent of the receptors are blocked. A post-tetanic twitch can be used to determine the reversibility of the block. Double burst stimulation can be used to moniter recovery from neuromuscular block.

Temperature measurement

It is important to be able to measure skin and core temperature during general anaesthesia. A variety of small thermistor temperature probes are available which give a digital display

Equipment monitoring

Anaesthetic machines should always be checked thoroughly prior to use.

Oxygen failure warning

All anaesthetic machines should be fitted with an oxygen failure warning device. It should be simple, reliable, and activated automatically when the machine is brought into use. If the oxygen fails the device should automatically cut off anaesthetic gases and allow air to be entrained.

Delivered oxygen concentration

Continuous monitoring of the delivered oxygen concentration using an in-line oxygen analyser is desirable. Polarographic or fuel cell devices are used. The upper and lower alarm limits should be set at 25 per cent and 40 per cent respectively to detect hypoxic mixtures, nitrous oxide failure, or an oxygen flush inadvertently left on. The device should be placed in the expiratory limb of the circuit, where the oxygen concentration should be within 3 per cent of the inspired concentration.

Measurement of volatile anaesthetic concentration
Monitoring of inspired and expired volatile anaesthetic concentrations is particularly important if low flow anaesthesia is being used.

Pressure monitoring
Pressure relief valves are included in all anaesthetic machines and breathing systems to prevent high pressures being delivered to the equipment or the patient. A pressure relief valve distal to the vaporizers is set at 35 kPa to prevent back-pressure if the outflow of the machine is occluded. A spring-loaded valve in the breathing system allows gas to escape when the pressure reaches 50 cm water (3–4 kPa), but it can be overridden. A disconnect alarm must be used if a patient is mechanically ventilated.

Gas volume measurement
It is vital to be able to measure gas volumes as well as composition and pressure. A respirometer must be available to measure inspired and expired gas volumes.

Minimum monitoring in the A & E department
Guidelines stress the importance of carbon dioxide monitoring and pulse oximetry. Oxygen supply monitoring and a pressure alarm warning of disconnection during mechanical ventilation are mandatory. The adoption of minimum standards of monitoring has medico-legal as well as safety implications. The following are suggested as minimum standards for monitoring equipment in the A & E department:

- Continuous clinical monitoring by a trained anaesthetist with an assistant
- All equipment familiar to anaesthetist, checked, and calibrated
- Continuous cardiorespiratory monitoring from induction of anaesthesia until full recovery
- Oxygen supply failure alarm
- Disconnect alarm if ventilator used

- High pressure warning alarm
- ECG monitoring
- Capnography
- Pulse oximetry
- Expiratory volume measurement available
- Means to measure temperature available

Emergency general anaesthesia – prehospital care

Initial patient management should follow the 'ABC' of resuscitation within the limitations of the environment. Life-threatening conditions should be treated. Very occasionally, it may be necessary to give an anaesthetic to allow amputation of a trapped limb and extrication of the patient. Much more commonly a trapped patient can be released by the fire brigade, using cutting or lifting equipment. Analgesia and intravenous fluids are often needed. All patients should be labelled with the name, dose, and timing of any drugs which they receive.

Ketamine

In the rare occasions when out-of-hospital anaesthesia is needed ketamine is the most appropriate drug to use. Ketamine is non-irritant and may be given intramuscularly or intravenously. About one-sixth of patients will have unpleasant emergent dreams.

Ketamine has the following advantages and limitations when used in prehospital care:

- It preserves the protective glottal reflexes more than other anaesthetic induction agents, although loss of airway competence is always a risk.

- It is probably the safest agent to use if the patient has a full stomach, although it does not protect against regurgitation.

- It stimulates the cardiovascular system and should therefore be used with caution in the head injured patient.

- Respiratory depression does not usually occur with normal clinical doses.
- It has a powerful analgesic action in sub-anaesthetic doses.
- Patients are easy to manage postoperatively. They are pain-free, travel well, and require minimal supervision.
- It has a shelf life of several years and does not need refrigeration; but it may deteriorate in temperatures of over 30°C.

Dosage and administration

Ketamine is supplied in three strengths: 10 mg/ml, 50 mg/ml, and 100 mg/ml. Ketamine may be used in pre-hospital care by non-anaesthetists with adequate training. Full anaesthetic dosage should only be given by anaesthetists, except in the most exceptional circumstances. Doses of ketamine which provide surgical anaesthesia are:

- *Intravenous*: 1–2 mg/kg. This should be given slowly over one minute. It becomes effective after 2–7 minutes, providing surgical anaesthesia for 5–10 minutes. The patient recovers from sleep after about 20 minutes.

- *Intramuscular*: 5–10 mg/kg. This becomes effective after 4–15 minutes, providing surgical anaesthesia for 12–25 minutes. The patient recovers from sleep after about one hour. Further doses may be given to prolong anaesthesia or to reduce the increased muscle tone which sometimes occurs with ketamine, and may be a hindrance during extrication.

- Repeat doses may be given as 10–20 mg intravenously; and 20–50 mg intramuscularly. Large limb movement is a useful sign that more ketamine is needed. Opening the eyes, looking around, or phonating are normal, and do not indicate the need for more ketamine. The eyes should be protected from foreign bodies if they remain open. Opioids may prolong the action of ketamine.

Special caution

Alcoholics do not settle well with ketamine. Psychotic patients may also respond badly. In an emergency these problems may not be considered as major contraindications. The use of a small dose of midazolam may minimize these problems. Ketamine raises blood pressure and should be avoided where possible in head injured patients or those known to be hypertensive. It is a bronchodilator and may be used in asthmatics. Overdose causes respiratory depression, but should not produce any long term problem so long as adequate ventilation can be maintained.

Further reading

Association of Anaesthetists of Great Britain and Ireland (1994). *Recommendations for standards of monitoring during anaesthesia and recovery*. A A G B I, London.

Cormack, R. S. and Lehane, J. (1984). Difficult intubation in obstetric anaesthesia. *Anaesthesia*, **39** , 1105–11.

Crosby, W. M. (1988). Checking anaesthetic machines, drugs and monitoring devices. *Anaesthesia and Intensive Care*, **16**, 32–4.

Dull, D. L., Tinker, J. H., Caplan, R. A., Ward, R. J., and Cheney, F. W. (1989). ASA closed claims study: can pulse oximetry and capnography prevent anaesthetic mishaps? *Anesthesia and Analgesia*, **68**, 574.

Eichorn, J. H., Cooper, J. B., Cullen, D. J., Maier, W. R., Philip, J. H., and Seeman, R. G. (1986). Standards for patient monitoring during anaesthesia at Harvard Medical School. *Journal of the American Medical Association*, **256**, 1017–20.

Mallampati, S. R., Gatt, S. P., and Gugino, L. D. (1985). A clinical sign to predict difficult tracheal intubation: a prospective study. *Canadian Anaesthetists Society Journal*, **32**, 429–34.

Stoneham, M. D. (1996). Anaesthesia for cardioversion. *Anaesthesia*, **51**, 565–70.

Sykes, M. K. (1987). Essential monitoring. *British Journal of Anaesthesia*, **59**, 901–12.

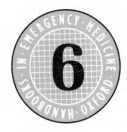

CHAPTER 6

Recovery and street fitness

Key points in recovery and street fitness

- The speed of initial recovery from general anaesthesia is due to drug redistribution. It bears little relationship to elimination of anaesthetic and sedative drugs. Some intravenous agents have active metabolites which can cause sedation after discharge from hospital.

- Sedatives and anaesthetic drugs may impair psychomotor skills. Studies have shown reductions in performance after outpatient anaesthesia.

- After anaesthesia or sedation patients must be looked after in a dedicated, properly staffed recovery area.

- The anaesthetist must stay with the patient until he or she responds to commands, protective reflexes have returned, and breathing and circulation are stable.

- Patients should remain in hospital under supervision for at least two hours after general anaesthesia. Fitness for discharge should be decided by a qualified person.

- The patient must be given verbal and written instructions on postoperative care, and arrangements for follow-up.

- Every patient going home should be looked after by a responsible adult.

- Adequate analgesia should be provided.

Anaesthesia and sedation in the A & E department must ensure optimal operating conditions and prompt, adequately supervised recovery. Similar considerations apply to recovery from anaesthesia and to sedation, as the boundary between the two states is blurred. The speed of initial recovery is due to drug redistribution. It bears little relationship to the complete elimination of anaesthetic and sedative drugs. Some intravenous agents have active metabolites which can cause sedation after discharge from hospital.

Assessment of recovery

The difficulty in evaluation of recovery is evident from the number of psychomotor tests available. These tests can detect residual effects of anaesthetic and sedative drugs. The Steward scoring system awards a score of 0, 1, or 2 points to each of three attributes, wakefulness, ventilation, and movement. Patients should only be discharged from hospital when they have attained a score of 6. The Maddox wing test can be used to assess the residual effects of sedation by measuring the balance of extraocular muscles to detect the degree of heterophoria. The 'critical flicker fusion' test measures the patient's ability to distinguish discrete sensory data as an index of central nervous system efficiency; it is a sensitive test of cognitive function following anaesthesia. Performance can be assessed by using the 'choice reaction time' apparatus. The patient places a finger on a rest template, and has to press a button in response to a light stimulus. The reaction recognition time (RRT) is the time taken to lift the hand from the template, and the total reaction time (TRT) is the time to reach the appropriate response button (the motor response time is calculated by TRT minus RRT. Tracking tests allow patients to track an arrow on a microcomputer screen using a joystick and respond to stimuli. Deviation from the track programme and reaction time can be derived. Body sway can be measured using an ataxiameter on patients standing with closed eyes. Tests of orientation, concentration, and memory can be used to assess recovery, for example, tests of deleting a particular letter from a passage of text, remembering a sequence of digits, or joining a series of dots.

Psychomotor tests are mainly used for research. They allow analysis of the more subtle effects of sedatives and anaesthetics which may be clinically important. The sensitivity of different tests and the implications of deviations from normal values are not clear. However, many studies have shown that patients may have a reduction in psycho-motor performance when they are discharged from hospital after outpatient anaesthesia. Alcohol, even in high doses, has little effect on psychomotor performance, even though psychomotor tests have a high sensitivity for other centrally acting drugs. Sedatives and anaesthetic drugs may therefore cause a more significant impairment of skills than alcohol; but warnings about these agents are often less stringent and less strictly enforced.

Postoperative recovery rooms

Appreciation of the importance of respiratory and cardiovas-cular complications after anaesthesia and surgery resulted in the introduction of postoperative recovery rooms in Britain over thirty years ago. The College and the Association of Anaesthetists recommend that patients are cared for in a dedicated, adequately staffed recovery area following anaes-thesia or sedation. The staff should be trained nurses or operating department personnel. The staff–patient ratio must be one to one. The staff must have no other duties whilst looking after a recovering patient. The recovery area must have tipping trolleys, suction apparatus, oxygen, and resuscitation equipment. Minimum available monitoring should include an ECG monitor, apparatus to measure blood pressure, a simple temperature monitor, capnograph, and pulse oximetry. Equipment maintenance should be clearly assigned. Drugs for treatment of cardiorespiratory collapse, anaphylaxis, bronchospasm, and hypoglycaemia should be immediately available. There should be easy access to anal-gesics and antiemetics. A written record of the patient's progress during the recovery period must be made, includ-ing any drugs administered. The anaesthetist must remain with the patient until protective reflexes have returned, the patient responds to command, and cardiorespiratory parameters are stable.

Problems during recovery

Twenty per cent of patients have problems during recovery from anaesthesia:

- Regurgitation and aspiration of gastric contents while protective reflexes are depressed, especially after trauma.
- Emesis, especially after opioids. Prompt treatment with intravenous antiemetics is necessary, as this may delay discharge from hospital.
- Airway obstruction: this may be due to bad head position, a foreign body (including a poorly placed oropharyngeal airway), or laryngospasm.
- Bronchospasm.
- Cardiovascular collapse due to an adverse drug reaction, cardiac arrhythmia, cardiac failure, unsuspected pneumothorax, or bleeding.
- Hypertension: this may be due to pain or hypoxaemia (or rarely phaeochromocytoma).
- Hyperthermia: this may be due to sepsis, hypermetabolism, or malignant hyperthermia.
- Confusion during emergence: this may be due to drugs, fear, or pain. However, hypoxaemia must always be considered. More sinister central nervous system problems may also lead to confusion (hypoglycaemia, ischaemia, or head injury).
- Slow recovery: this may be due to drugs (taken before or given during anaesthesia or sedation), hypoxaemia, hypocapnia, hypotension, or incidental causes, such as central nervous system problems (stroke or head injury), metabolic problems (electrolyte disturbance, uraemia, liver disease, or hypoglycaemia), or endocrine disease (hypopituitary, hypothyroid, or hypoadrenal states). Any patient who recovers significantly more slowly than anticipated should be admitted to hospital for overnight observation.

Discharge from hospital

Patients should remain in hospital under supervision for at least 2 hours after anaesthesia. A qualified person should decide when a patient is fit for discharge from hospital. The operation site must be checked before the patient is discharged from hospital. The patients should be able to hold a sensible conversation and walk unaided (assuming the surgical procedure allows). The patient must be given verbal and written instructions. He or she should be accompanied and subsequently looked after by a responsible person (not an infirm relative or a child). The patient should be instructed not to drive, climb ladders, operate machinery, use dangerous household appliances (for example a cooker), look after children, drink alcohol, take other sedatives, or make important decisions for 24–48 hours after the procedure. Advice about postoperative care and arrangements for any follow up attendance should be given in writing. Adequate simple analgesia should be provided.

Further reading

Association of Anaesthetists of Great Britain and Ireland (1985). *Post-anaesthetic recovery facilities.* AAGBI, London.

Fagan, D., Tiplady, B., and Scott, D. B. (1987). Effects of ethanol on psychomotor performance. *British Journal of Anaesthesia,* **59,** 961–5.

Hannington-Kiff, J. G. (1970). Measurement of recovery from outpatient general anaesthesia with a simple ocular test. *British Medical Journal,* **3,** 132.

Hindmarsh, I. (1982). Critical flicker fusion frequency (CFFF); the effects of psychotropic compounds. *Pharmacopsychiatrica,* **15,** (Suppl. 1), 44.

Hindmarsh, I. and Subhan, Z. (1983). The effects of midazolam in conjunction with alcohol on sleep, psychomotor performance and car driving ability. *International Journal of Clinical Pharmacology Research,* **3,** 323.

Hindmarch, I., Subhan, Z., and Stoker, M. (1983). The effects of amitriptyline on car driving and psychomotor performance. *Acta Psychiatrica Scandinavica,* **68** (Suppl. 308), 141.

Steward, D. J. (1975). A simplified scoring system for the postoperative recovery room. *Canadian Anaesthetists Society Journal,* **22,** 111–13.

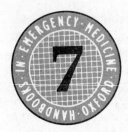

CHAPTER 7

Problems encountered during general anaesthesia

Key points in problems encountered during general anaesthesia

- All problems occurring during anaesthesia must be managed logically and systematically. Assessment and treatment of priorities as airway, breathing, and circulation ('ABC') is fundamental to safe practice.
- The response to a problem partly depends upon the experience of the anaethetist. It is important to have adequate trained assistance and to summon senior help quickly.
- Careful preoperative assessment often predicts potential difficulties.
- In the event of a problem, it is important to communicate with the patient, their carers, and other staff afterwards. In some circumstances, it is essential to inform the patient's general practitioner of the situation.

It is essential to manage problems which occur during anaesthesia logically and systematically. The priorities of 'airway, breathing, and circulation' – ABC – are fundamental to safe practice in all situations. The response to a problem depends upon the patient's condition and the experience of the anaesthetist. It is vital to have adequate trained assistance and to summon senior help quickly. Careful preoperative assessment often predicts potential difficulties, for example intubation problems or a family history of malignant hyperthermia. Other difficulties are unpredictable and the anaesthetist must have a simple plan of action for each situation. The basic way of dealing with any problem is to address airway, breathing, and circulation and then find the cause of the problem and treat it specifically. It is important to communicate with the patient, their carers, and other staff afterwards. In some circumstances it is essential to inform the patient's general practitioner of the situation, for example after a hypersensitivity reaction or suxamethonium apnoea.

Cardiovascular problems

Cardiac arrest

Pallor, absent major pulses, unrecordable blood pressure, diminishing end-tidal carbon dioxide concentration, and falling transcutaneous oxygen saturation signal cardiac arrest. The ECG may show asystole or ventricular fibrillation, or electromechanical dissociation.

Causes
- Hypoxaemia
- Hypotension
- Cardiac event, for example progression of cardiac arrhythmia, myocardial infarction, or cardiac tamponade
- A ventilatory problem, for example pneumothorax
- Electrolyte or acid–base disturbance
- Drug overdose or allergy
- A central nervous system problem, for example cerebral bleeding or raised intracranial pressure

Treatment
1. Call for help and place the patient supine on a hard surface.
2. Follow the recommendations of the Resuscitation Council of the United Kingdom for defibrillation and drug administration (see p. 126).
3. Treat specific problems appropriately.

Bradycardia and bradyarrhythmias

Sinus bradycardia is defined as a pulse rate of less than 60 beats per minute in an adult. Young children have much faster heart rates, and a rate of 80 beats per minute may represent significant bradycardia in an infant. A bradycardia which is not sinus often indicates a serious problem and may progress to asystole.

Causes

- Hypoxaemia. Bradycardia is a late sign of inadequate oxygenation in adults, but occurs early in children.
- Vagal stimulation, such as intubation and carotid sinus pressure. Light anaesthesia may potentiate vagal over-activity.
- Drugs, for example suxamethonium, digoxin, beta blockers, halothane, opioids, or neostigmine.
- Physiological bradycardia is common in athletic young people.
- A cardiac problem, such as ischaemia or heart block.
- Raised intracranial pressure.
- Hypothermia.
- Hypothyroidism.

Treatment

Treatment is needed if bradycardia compromises cardiac output or seems likely to progress to a more serious condition. Young patients, the elderly, and those with a fixed cardiac output should be treated early, as they may not maintain an adequate circulation if the heart rate is too slow.

1. Ensure adequate oxygenation of the patient.
2. If anaesthesia is too light, deepen the level and ask the surgeon to stop stimulating the patient until control is achieved.
3. If there are no other remediable causes, administer atropine intravenously (adult 0.6–1.0 mg, child 0.02 mg/kg).
4. If bradycardia persists, or is not sinus, consider the use of isoprenaline intravenously (1.5 µg/kg bolus or 0.01–0.1

μg/kg/min.). Temporary cardiac pacing may be needed, especially in complete heart block, second degree heart block, symptomatic first degree heart block, trifascicular block, and sick sinus syndrome.

Tachycardia, ventricular ectopic beats, and tachyarrhythmias

Sinus tachycardia is defined as a heart rate of more than 100 beats per minute in an adult. Neonates and infants have much faster resting heart rates. Supraventricular or ventricular arrhythmias may be seen.

Causes
- Hypoxaemia
- Hypercapnia
- Hypovolaemia and hypotension (which must be corrected prior to anaesthesia)
- Light anaesthesia, awarenesss
- Drugs such as atropine, halothane, adrenaline, or some inotropes
- Glucose, electrolyte, or acid–base disturbance
- Cardiac problems
- Hyperthermia
- Thyrotoxicosis
- Adverse reaction to blood or drugs
- Catecholamine-secreting tumour

Treatment
1. Ensure that oxygenation, ventilation, and the circulating volume of the patient are adequate.
2. Treat sinus tachycardia if it is an inappropriate response or if it comprises cardiac output or myocardial oxygenation.
3. Deepen anaesthesia if the patient is too lightly anaesthetized, but otherwise well.
4. Discontinue any drugs which may exacerbate the problem.
5. Measure and correct the plasma electrolytes.

6. Supraventricular tachycardia should be treated if the cause cannot be addressed and cardiac output is reduced. Antiarrhythmic drugs are all negative inotropes which may impair cardiac performance. Supraventricular tachycardia may respond to carotid sinus massage, adenosine (adult dose 3mg doubling dose until effective), or verapamil (75–150 µg/kg). Atrial fibrillation may respond to digoxin (3.5–7.0 µg/kg loading dose). Fast atrial fibrillation of recent onset may be treated with flecainide (initial dose 2mg/kg). DC cardioversion may be needed if there is circulatory compromise.

7. Ventricular tachycardias should be treated intravenously using lignocaine 0.5–3.0 mg/kg, and/or defibrillation.

8. Arrhythmias due to local anaesthetic toxicity may be treated with bretylium 7mg/kg followed by an infusion.

Hypertension

Hypertension during anaesthesia is usually due to increased peripheral vascular resistance. Hypertension should be diagnosed with reference to the patient's normal blood pressure. The width of the blood pressure cuff must be at least two-thirds of the length of the upper arm. Small cuffs may give a falsely high reading, especially on large arms. Paediatric cuffs must be used in children.

Causes
• Hypoxaemia or hypercarbia
• Pre-existing hypertension
• Stimulation of the patient causing catecholamine release, such as laryngoscopy or surgery under light anaesthesia
• Drugs such as ergometrine, cocaine, or adrenaline
• Phaeochromocytoma
• Eclampsia
• Raised intracranial pressure

Treatment
1. Ensure that the patient is adequately oxygenated and ventilated.

2. If the patient is too lightly anaesthetized, reduce the

stimulation, if possible, until the patient is more deeply anaesthetized.

3. If hypertension reaches dangerous levels treat with specific drugs such as labetolol or esmolol, sublingual nifedipine (10–20 mg in an adult), hydralazine (up to 0.3 mg/kg), or nitroglycerine (0.8–2.0 µg/kg/min). Particular care must be taken to control blood pressure in patients with cardiac or cerebrovascular problems.

Hypotension

Hypotension may be due to a fall in peripheral vascular resistance or a decrease in cardiac output. The pulse pressure narrows when cardiac output falls. Autoregulation may not compensate for severe hypotension in patients with vascular disease. Brain, cardiac, and renal perfusion may be compromised if hypotension persists. Severe hypotension may progress to cardiac arrest.

Causes
- Hypoxaemia
- Hypercapnia
- Hypovolaemia
- Anaesthetic drugs, most of which decrease peripheral vascular resistance, and some of which reduce cardiac output
- Histamine release, which commonly occurs after thiopentone, atropine, opioids, and some muscle relaxants
- Anaphylactoid reaction
- Sympathetic block by local anaesthetics
- Posture, such as head-up tilt or aorto-caval compression
- Intermittent positive pressure ventilation
- Reduced cardiac output, due to cardiac arrhythmias, electrolyte or acid–base problems, negative inotropes, heart failure, cardiac tamponade, or pneumothorax
- Sepsis

Treatment
1. Ensure adequate oxygenation and ventilation of the patient, try to keep the airway inflation pressures as low as feasible.

2. Establish regular measurement of oxygen saturation, heart rate, and blood pressure.

3. Organize venous access.

4. Elevate the patient's legs if possible and reduce any aorto-caval compression.

5. Reduce the use of anaesthetic and negatively inotropic drugs as much as is practical.

6. Find the cause of hypotension. Treat hypovolaemia with intravenous fluid boluses (20 ml/kg initially). Treat cardiac failure with inotropes such as dopamine or dobutamine (2–10 μg/kg/min.). Dopexamine is an inotrope without vasoconstrictor activity which may be useful in some situations. Cardiac failure associated with vasodilatation, such as septic shock, may need treatment with inotropes such as noradrenaline 4–12 μg/kg/min or adrenaline 1–4 μg/min (adult doses).

7. If hypotension is due to sympathetic blockade, administer increments of intravenous ephedrine, up to a maximum of 30 mg in an adult.

8. Decide whether invasive monitoring is needed to establish the diagnosis and direct treatment.

Major bleeding

Major haemorrhage under anaesthesia is dangerous because the patient's ability to compensate by vasoconstriction is reduced.

Causes
- Disease or trauma
- Surgery
- Coagulopathy

Treatment
1. Administer 100 per cent oxygen.

2. Establish venous access with two large-bore peripheral cannulae. Only use central venous access if peripheral cannulation is impossible and the practitioner is experienced in the technique. Intraosseous infusion may be useful in children with difficult veins.

3. Send blood for type and cross-matching. Fully cross-matched blood is preferable, but this may take an hour to be available. Most transfusion services can provide type-specific or 'saline cross-matched' blood in 10–15 minutes. This blood is compatible with ABO and Rhesus blood types, but may be incompatible with minor antibodies. It may be used in those with life-threatening haemorrhage who cannot wait for fully cross-matched blood. If type-specific blood is not available, and the patient is exsanguinating, type O Rhesus negative packed cells can be given. Microfilters should not be used as these are of no proven benefit and slow the infusion rate. All fluids must be warmed.

4. Administer 20 ml/kg crystalloid initially. Observe the response and then administer colloid or blood appropriately.

5. Establish invasive monitoring if necessary, but do not allow this to delay active management of the problem.

6. Insert a urinary catheter.

7. If the patient has received a massive blood transfusion, check the coagulation and treat appropriately. Calcium administration is not indicated and may be harmful.

Respiratory problems

Airway problems

It is sometimes possible to anticipate that airway maintenance or intubation may be difficult in a particular patient. It is important to have all the aids to promote good airway control checked and within reach. Fibre-optic intubation is useful but requires practice and experience. It should never be used in an emergency situation for the first time. Skilled assistance is vital during induction, maintenance, and recovery from anaesthesia. The most important rule is that a patient with a difficult airway must never be given a muscle relaxant until the anaesthetist is certain that it is possible to oxygenate the patient adequately.

Causes

- Congenital or acquired facial deformity. Protruding teeth, receding jaw, overbite, or high arched palate are warning signs.
- Reduced mouth opening due to trismus or deformity.
- Difficulty with neck movement (especially poor atlanto-occipital joint extension) or an unstable cervical spine.
- Epiglottitis or laryngeal pathology; stridor is a very significant sign.
- Tracheal stenosis, compression, or deviation.
- Foreign body in the airway.
- Trauma.

Treatment

1. Never give elective anaesthesia in the A & E department to a patient with a difficult airway.
2. If the problem is only recognized after induction of anaesthesia try simple methods to improve the situation and concentrate on oxygenating the patient. Try to keep the patient breathing spontaneously. Good head position and the gentle use of a nasopharyngeal or oral airway may help. If manual ventilation is difficult, ask an assistant to squeeze the reservoir bag whilst using both hands to maintain the airway. If the airway is difficult to manage, the careful use of a laryngeal mask airway may help to provide oxygenation in some circumstances. It cannot protect the airway against aspiration, and must never be used with high inflation pressures.
3. If the airway remains difficult to maintain, abandon the procedure and wake the patient up, using the failed intubation drill (see p. 107).
4. If the airway is easy to maintain, but intubation is difficult, wake the patient up. It is not usually wise to proceed with elective surgery in a patient who cannot be intubated in the A & E department.
5. If intubation is needed, for example in an emergency situation, try cricoid pressure to displace the larynx backwards, the use of a gum-elastic bougie to direct the trachael tube, or blind nasal intubation in experienced

hands. If intubation fails, institute the failed intubation drill (see next section), and summon senior help.

6. Oesophageal intubation is fatal if it is not recognized. Definite ways to confirm intubation of the trachea are: to see the tube enter the vocal cords, to view the trachea via the tube using a fibre-optic instrument, and to detect a significant end-tidal carbon dioxide concentration emerging from the trachael tube for at least five ventilatory cycles.

Failed intubation drill

It is vital that all anaesthetists and their assistants are familiar with a failed intubation drill, which must be instituted when intubation attempts are abandoned. The most difficult decision is to give up trying to intubate a patient. Persistent futile attempts at intubation cause hypoxaemia and increase the risk of aspiration.

1. State that attempts at intubation are over, maintain cricoid pressure, and call for senior help.

2. Attempt to ventilate the patient with a face mask and an oral or nasal airway, using 100 per cent oxygen.

3. If ventilation is impossible, turn the patient 15 degrees to the left lateral and head-down position, keeping the cricoid pressure on to reduce the risk of aspiration.

4. If ventilation is still impossible, ask the assistant to slowly release the cricoid pressure, and try to ventilate again. If this is not possible a laryngeal mask airway may help, but should only be used by experienced staff.

5. If oxygenation is still impossible turn the patient back to the supine position. Perform either cricothyroid puncture with transtracheal ventilation or cricothyroidotomy and placement of a small diameter tracheal tube.

6. Allow the patient to wake up.

7. Once the patient has fully recovered, discuss the problem with a senior anaesthetist. Warn the patient if the intubation problem is likely to persist, make careful notes in the case records, and inform the patient's general practitioner about the situation.

Laryngospasm

Laryngospasm occurs when the intrinsic laryngeal muscles contract and occlude the glottis, preventing ventilation and resulting in hypoxaemia.

Causes
- Stimulation of the patient during light anaesthesia
- Irritant vapours
- Airway irritation by secretions, vomit, blood, or an airway
- Extubation of a lightly anaesthetized patient

Treatment
1. Administer 100 per cent oxygen (experienced anaesthetists may opt to deepen anaesthesia in some situations).
2. Clear the airway; use the suction gently.
3. Ventilate the patient with positive pressure. Try not to inflate the stomach, as this increases the risk of regurgitation.
4. In severe laryngospasm consider the use of suxamethonium but only if the patient is known to be easy to ventilate manually. If suxamethonium is given to a hypoxaemic patient, bradycardia requiring the use of atropine may occur.
5. Mild laryngospasm may respond to 0.1 mg/kg suxametronium, which will work within 2 minutes.
6. Intubation is occasionally needed.

Bronchospasm

In a patient who is breathing spontaneously bronchospasm may be manifested by difficulty with breathing, prolonged expiration, and the use of accessory muscles of respiration. In a ventilated patient it may be revealed by difficulty in inflating the patient's chest or a rise in airway pressure. Wheezing may be heard on auscultation; but in severe cases, if no gas entry is possible, the chest may be silent. If bronchospasm is severe hypoxaemia and hypercapnia occur, often precipitating cardiac arrhythmias.

Causes
- Asthma or chronic obstructive airway disease
- Smoking
- Irritation of the airway by oropharyngeal airways, tracheal tubes, or irritant volatile agents
- Surgical stimulation during light anaesthesia
- Predictable reactions to drugs such as beta blockers and histamine releasers
- Anaphylactoid reaction

Treatment
1. Check that the patient has bronchospasm and not upper airway obstruction or a misplaced tracheal tube. Make sure that the upper airway is completely clear.
2. Observe the transcutaneous oxygen saturation. It may be necessary to give 100 per cent oxygen to maintain oxygen.
3. Decide whether to wake the patient up or to maintain deep anaesthesia. Do not allow stimulation of a lightly anaesthetized patient. Volatile anaesthetic agents all dilate bronchi, but pungent agents may initially worsen bronchospasm.
4. Give a bronchodilator, such as aminophylline 5 mg/kg (if the patient is not already taking theophyllines) or salbutamol (3 μg/kg), by slow intravenous injection, with careful observation of the ECG monitor. Nebulized racemic adrenaline (1mg L-adrenaline in 5ml saline) may be used.
5. Severe bronchspasm or anaphylaxis require the use of adrenaline 5–10 μg intravenously, repeated as often as necessary up to 500 μg or given in a 0.01–0.3 μg/kg/min infusion. The tracheal route has limited application in patients with bronchospasm.
6. When high airway-inflation pressures are needed there is always a risk of pneumothorax and mediastinal emphysema.

Pneumothorax

A small pneumothorax may be difficult to detect clinically, and the diagnosis may depend on the history of the problem.

A tension pneumothorax may be apparent on clinical examination of the chest when the trachea is deviated away from the affected side, where the chest is hyperresonant and breath sounds are reduced. When the patient is breathing spontaneously a pneumothorax may gradually increase in size and compromise gas exchange. If a patient is manually ventilated, especially with nitrous oxide, a tension pneumothorax may develop quickly. Bilateral pneumothoraces are life threatening and must be remedied immediately.

Causes
- Air may enter the pleural cavity as a result of trauma, surgery, the insertion of central lines, brachial plexus block, and the use of high airway inflation pressures
- Asthmatic patients and those with emphysematous bullae are especially at risk
- Positive pressure ventilation and nitrous oxide may worsen a pneumothorax

Treatment
1. Maintain oxygenation of the patient.
2. Stop use of nitrous oxide.
3. Make the diagnosis of pneumothorax clinically, there is often no time for X-ray confirmation. Urgent drainage is needed if the patient is ventilated or has a large expanding pneumothorax. Insert a wide-bore cannula through the second intercostal space in the mid-clavicular line. If there is an escape of air the patient should improve quickly. A chest drain should then be inserted in the fifth intercostal space anterior to the midaxillary line on the affected side. It should be connected to a one way valve or an underwater drainage bottle. If a one-way valve is used, care should be taken to ensure that it is connected correctly and does not become blocked.
4. If a patient with a pneumothorax does not improve after insertion of a chest drain, check that the drain is patent. Consider needle thoracentesis and drainage of the contralateral side.
5. Elective chest drains may be needed prior to anaesthesia in patients with chest trauma.

Hypoxaemia

Central cyanosis is seen when there is more than 5 g/dl of reduced haemoglobin present. Severe anaemia may mask cyanosis, and polycythaemia may make it more apparent. Clinical observation of cyanosis can be difficult in patients with pigmented skin; but transcutaneous monitoring of oxygen saturation is independent of skin colour. Reduced oxygen saturation is an indication of inadequate tissue oxygenation and action must be taken to rectify the situation immediately.

Causes

- Delivery of a gas mixture with a low oxygen concentration to the patient, or disconnection of the anaesthetic circuit
- Obstructed airway
- Bronchospasm or pneumothorax
- Apnoea or hypoventilation
- Pulmonary oedema
- Decreased lung blood flow, due for example to heart failure, pulmonary embolus, or collapsed lung
- Increased oxygen demand, due for example to malignant hyperthermia or thyrotoxicosis
- Inability of the cells to utilize oxygen

Treatment

1. Check that the oxygen analyser on the anaesthetic equipment is showing the required inspired oxygen concentration and that the pulse oximeter is correctly placed and accurate. Check that the anaesthetic equipment is working correctly.

2. Increase the inspired oxygen concentration whilst assessing the problem and verify that the oxygen analyser responds to the change. If using a low flow system change to a higher flow.

3. In a spontaneously breathing patient confirm that the airway is clear and that the patient is breathing. Gently attempt to ventilate the patient manually with 100 per cent oxygen.

4. Look for problems with the airway. End-tidal carbon dioxide detection verifies placement of the tracheal tube. If there is doubt about a laryngeal mask or tracheal tube it must be removed. The patient must be oxygenated until it is replaced.

5. Examine the patient's chest for endobronchial intubation, bronchospasm, collapsed lung, pulmonary oedema, or pneumothorax. Treat appropriately.

6. Ensure that the patient has adequate pulse and blood pressure.

7. If a cause cannot quickly be found and remedied, summon senior help and terminate the anaesthetic as promptly as is feasible.

8. Measure core temperature.

Inability to ventilate an intubated patient

If an intubated patient develops a high airway pressure or cannot be ventilated manually the anaesthetist must make a rapid systematic assessment of the problem.

Causes
- A blocked tracheal tube, caused for example by kinking, a foreign body, biting by the patient, a herniated cuff, or the tube being pushed against the tracheal wall or carina
- A more proximal obstruction, for example in the valve system, or the catheter mount or circuit.
- A more distal obstruction, for example due to a foreign body in the airway, lung collapse, bronchospasm, pulmonary oedema, or pneumothorax
- Coughing, struggling, or chest wall rigidity

Treatment
1. Administer 100 per cent oxygen.
2. If the patient is being ventilated mechanically, change to manual ventilation.
3. If there is doubt about the circuit proximal to the tracheal tube, disconnect the circuit and use a self-inflating bag with supplementary oxygen.

4. Check the tracheal tube, try to ventilate with the cuff deflated, and use a suction catheter to investigate the possibility of a blockage. If there is ANY doubt remove the tube and ventilate with a bag and mask system.

5. Examine the chest to diagnose lung collapse, pulmonary oedema, bronchospasm, or pneumothorax.

Aspiration of gastric contents into the lungs

Any patient at risk of aspiration of gastric contents must not be given elective anaesthesia in the A & E department. In an emergency situation the use of a rapid sequence anaesthetic induction technique is mandatory. Any patient who may have aspirated must be admitted to hospital for observation.

Causes
- A full stomach, for example following a recent meal, trauma, diabetic ketoacidosis, the use of opioids, swallowed blood after trauma, surgery, or gastrointestinal pathology
- Women in the third trimester of pregnancy are particularly at risk
- High intragastric pressure due to obesity, pressure on the abdomen, or gases entering the stomach during manual ventilation
- Difficulty with airway management increases the risk of aspiration, especially during instrumentation of the pharynx or larynx during light anaesthesia

Treatment
1. If a patient regurgitates during induction of anaesthesia apply cricoid pressure, clear the airway using suction, position the patient head-down and on the left side, and intubate as rapidly as possible. If intubation is not possible follow the failed intubation drill (see p. 107).

2. After intubation use a suction catheter to apply endo-bronchial suction prior to manual ventilation with 100 per cent oxygen. Do not use saline bronchial lavage, as it spreads the contamination.

3. Examine the chest to detect collapse or bronchospasm; the patient may need bronchoscopy or bronchodilators.

4. Monitor the transcutaneous oxygen saturation, and measure blood gases if hypoxaemia occurs.

5. Antibiotics and steroids are not first line treatment.

6. Consult a senior anaesthetist, and transfer the patient to a high dependency or intensive care facility.

Tachypnoea

A cause should be sought for a respiratory rate faster than 20 breaths per minute in an adult. Rates of more than 40 breaths per minute in an infant and 60 breaths per minute in a neonate are significant.

Causes
- Severe hypoxaemia
- Hypercapnia
- Light anaesthesia
- Chest problems, such as infection or aspiration of gastric contents
- Metabolic problems, such as acidosis in diabetes, shock, or renal failure
- Pyrexia, due for example to infection or malignant hyperthermia

Treatment
1. Check for hypoxaemia, and increase the inspired oxygen concentration if necessary.
2. Assist ventilation to correct any hypercapnia.
3. Assess the chest clinically.
4. Measure temperature.
5. Evaluate acid–base status.
6. Deepen anaesthesia if it is deemed to be too light and no other cause can be found for tachypnoea. Remember that some volatile anaestesics can cause tacchycardia.

Apnoea

If a patient stops breathing after induction of anaesthesia or during surgery the cause may be related to the anaesthesia and/or the surgery, or it may be a separate problem.

Causes
- An airway problem, for example obstruction or aspiration of gastric contents.
- Ventilatory depression due to hypocarbia or drugs
- Surgical stimulation during light anaesthesia
- Cardiac arrest
- A central nervous system problem, for example stroke

Treatment
1. Examine the airway and ventilate the patient manually.
2. Ensure that oxygenation and the circulation of the patient are adequate.
3. Adjust the depth of anaesthesia appropriately and ask the surgeon to stop operating if necessary.
4. Adjust ventilation to achieve normocapnia.
5. Look for signs of a systemic problem.

Central nervous system problems

Fitting

It is unusual for a patient to have a fit during a general anaesthetic. Fitting may occur during the recovery period.

Causes
- Epilepsy
- Drugs such as methohexitone, enflurane, or propofol
- Hypoglycaemia
- Cerebral ischaemia or tumour
- Local anaesthetic toxicity
- Eclampsia

Treatment
1 Administer 100 per cent oxygen.
2. Maintain control of the airway.
3. Check that the patient has a palpable pulse.
4. Withdraw any drugs which may promote seizures and avoid hyperventilation of the patient.

5. Measure the blood glucose and treat hypoglycaemia.
6. If convulsions persist administer intravenous Diazemuls up to 0.3 mg/kg or thiopentone 3.5–5.0 mg/kg. Thiopentone may cause apnoea and should only be administered by staff who are confident in airway management. If convulsions persist it may be necessary to institute treatment with phenytoin by slow intravenous infusion, repeated after 30 minutes if necessary.
7. It may be necessary to paralyse and ventilate the patient to ensure adequate oxygenation. Paralysis does not stop seizure activity, which must be controlled by anticonvulsants.

Failure to regain consciousness after anaesthesia

A systematic assessment of the problem is essential.

Causes
- Continued action of drugs such as barbiturates, opioids, and benzodiazepines. Nitrous oxide and volatile agents usually wear off rapidly. Hepatic or renal problems may increase the duration of action of some anaesthetic drugs.
- Problems with ventilation. Hyperventilation reduces brain carbon dioxide concentration and decreases ventilatory drive. Hypoventilation produces severe hypercapnia and sedation.
- Hypoglycaemia.
- Cerebral problems due to hypotension, hypoxaemia, cerebral oedema, bleeding or infarction.
- Reduced thyroid, pituitary, or adrenal function.
- Hypothermia.
- Profound electrolyte disturbance.

Treatment
1. Check that the oxygenation and circulation of the patient are adequate.
2. Correct any abnormalities of arterial blood gases and acid–base status.
3. Check blood glucose and correct any problems.

4. Failure to regain consciousness due to central nervous problems must be differentiated from persistent paralysis by the use of a nerve stimulator.
5. Measure and correct the patient's temperature.
6. Consult a senior anaesthetist and transfer the patient to the intensive care unit.

Confusion

Any patient who becomes persistently confused following general anaesthesia must be admitted to hospital for observation.

Causes
- Effects of anaesthetic or analgesic drugs
- Elderly patients may become confused in hospital
- Hypoxaemia
- Hypoglycaemia
- Cerebral problems such as ischaemia, bleeding, or oedema
- Pain
- Psychiatric problem
- Alcohol or drug withdrawal

Treatment
1. If the patient is hypoxaemic administer oxygen by mask.
2. Correct any hypoglycaemia.
3. Assess pain control. Give analgesia or a nerve block if appropriate.
4. Examine the nervous system, look for localizing signs. Ask for a neurological or neurosurgical opinion if appropriate.
5. Ask for a psychiatric opinion if appropriate.

Awareness

It is possible for a paralysed patient to be inadequately anaesthetized and aware of their surroundings and the surgical procedure. It is a potential cause of litigation and requires sensitive handling and good communication with the patient.

Causes
- Failure to administer adequate anaesthesia, often during total intravenous technique
- Failure to observe for signs of awareness such as sweating, lachrymation, tachycardia, or hypertension
- Equipment failure, for example disconnection of the breathing circuit, air entrainment with dilution of anaesthetic gases, or accidental continuous activation of the oxygen flush

Treatment
1. The most important aspect of management of awareness is avoidance. Adequate anaesthesia is vital. Supplementation of intravenous techniques with volatile agents (with agent monitoring) decreases the chance of awareness. Careful equipment checking and maintenance are mandatory.
2. If awareness is suspected during a procedure immediately check the equipment and adjust the level of anaesthesia.
3. If awareness is suspected by the anaesthetist or reported by the patient a postoperative visit from the anaesthetist is important. The patient should be believed and treated sympathetically. The reason for the problem must be explained and documented in the case notes. The anaesthetist should try to reduce the patient's fear about anaesthetics. The patient should be told to discuss the problem with the anaesthetist if another anaesthetic is required in the future.

Muscle problems

Persistent paralysis after the use of a muscle relaxant

A transcutaneous nerve stimulator is essential to assess persistent paralysis following the use of a neuromuscular blocker (NMB).

Causes
- Continued effect of suxamethonium due to defective enzyme function

- Continued effect of NMB due to hepatic or renal problems, or failure to give an adequate dose of neostigmine
- Overdose of neostigmine
- Hypothermia
- Drug interactions leading to increased duration of NMB
- Some uncommon muscle diseases, for example myotonia and muscular dystrophy may lead to persistant weakness after NMBs.

Treatment

1. If paralysis persists, maintain anaesthesia and oxygenation.
2. Transfer the patient to an appropriate facility.
3. Wait for the effect of the muscle relaxant to wear off.
4. Do not administer more neostigmine or fresh frozen plasma.
5. Measure and type plasma cholinesterase and counsel the patient and family in cases of suxamenthonium apnoea.

Malignant hyperthermia

Malignant hyperthermia is a genetic muscle problem which is inherited as an autosomal dominant characteristic. The incidence is 1:200 000 in the United Kingdom, with a male:female ratio of 3:1. If there is hypoxaemia, hypercapnia, muscle rigidity, and a rise in core temperature of more than 2°C per hour, malignant hyperthermia must be considered. The differential diagnosis includes sepsis, posttransfusion pyrexia, a hypothalamic problem, hypermetabolism, hyperthyroidism, or phaeochromocytoma. The use of humidifiers, warming blankets, and blood warmers may cause hyperthermia, especially in children.

Causes

- Triggering anaesthetic drugs such as suxamethonium and volatile agents in susceptible individuals. A history of a previous uncomplicated anaesthetic involving triggering agents does not preclude malignant hyperthermia.

Treatment

1. Increase the inspired oxygen concentration to 100 per cent, remove triggering agents, and discontinue surgery as soon as feasible. Intravenous barbiturates or propofol and opioids can be used to maintain anaesthesia. Use an anaesthetic circuit which has not been in contact with volatile agents.

2. Monitor the heart rate, blood pressure, and core temperature accurately.

3. Discontinue all attempts to keep the patient warm. Begin active cooling, using surface cooling (ice packs over major arteries, fans, and a cooling blanket). Give cold intravenous fluids and cold bladder and gastric washouts, if the patient is intubated.

4. Give intravenous dantrolene 1–10 mg/kg.

5. Measure and correct arterial blood gases and acid–base balance. Measure plasma potassium and creatine kinase.

6. Transfer the patient to a high dependency or intensive care unit. Measure creatine kinase 6,12, and 24 hours after the reaction.

7. Encourage a diuresis to avoid obstructive renal failure due to myoglobin. Collect the first voided urine for measurement of myoglobin.

8. Subsequently refer the patient to the national screening unit in St James's University Hospital, Leeds.

Miscellaneous problems

Intra-arterial or subcutaneous injection of irritant substances

Intra-arterial injection of an irritant substance (such as thiopentone) is manifest by pain distal to the injection site and blanching of the tissues. Distal pulses may become poor-volume or absent. Subcutaneous injection of irritant agents may produce pain and/or tissue loss.

Treatment of intra-arterial injection
- Leave the needle in the artery

- Inject down the same needle with 10–20 ml plain procaine or 10–40 mg papaverine in 5–10 ml normal saline to try to dilate the artery
- Abandon the proposed procedure unless it is life saving
- Perform a sympathetic block of the limb using plain bupivacaine (stellate and brachial plexus block for the arm or lumbar sympathectomy for the leg)
- Consider the use of systemic anticoagulants
- Elevate the limb and provide analgesia
- Ask for the opinion of a vascular or reconstructive surgeon

Treatment of subcutaneous injection

1. Inject subcutaneously around the affected area with 3000 I U hyaluronidase in 10–20 ml normal saline to dilute the irritant.
2. Elevate the limb and provide analgesia.
3. Ask early for the opinion of a vascular or reconstructive surgeon if necessary.

Compartment syndrome

Compartment sydrome is due to increased tissue pressure within the confined spaces of the facial sheaths in limbs. The lower extremities are more often affected than the upper, especially the anterior tibial compartment. Compartment syndrome causes loss of integrity of the microcirculation with exudation of fluid into the interstitial spaces leading to oedema, muscle swelling, and raised compartmental pressure. When interstitial tissue pressure is greater than that in the capillary bed, local ischaemia with nerve and muscle injury occurs. Permanent paralysis and muscle necrosis may develop. Compartment syndrome usually develops over several hours. It can be suspected from the clinical history. Pain in the limb increased by muscle stretching and reduction in sensation are early signs. Tense swelling of the area and muscle weakness then develop. Vascular and neurological signs occur later. The diagnosis can be supported by measurement of tissue pressures within each compartment. Pressures of more than 35–45 mm Hg are suggestive of compartment syndrome. Regional anaesthetic techniques do not increase the risk of compartment syndrome BUT MAY MASK THE EARLY SIGNS.

Causes
- Trauma for example crush injury, open, or closed fractures
- Direct pressure, for example in a patient who has been lying unconscious and immobile for a prolonged period
- Reperfusion injury
- Drug or hyperosmolar fluid extravasation
- Malignant hyperthermia
- Prolonged use of pneumatic anti-shock garments

Treatment
1. Release any restrictive dressings.
2. Perform early fasciotomy of all affected compartments within 4 hours of development of the problem.
3. Support and elevate the limb.
4. Administer analgesia.
5. Refer the patient to a vascular or reconstructive surgeon.

Dental damage

The advice and help of an oral surgeon is invaluable in the event of dental trauma.

Causes
- Damage during airway maintenance, especially when the patient is lightly anaesthetized
- Damage during recovery

Treatment
1. Retrieve any teeth that are lost. If a tooth is missing a chest X-ray is mandatory, because an inhaled tooth may form a septic focus. Bronchoscopy is indicated to recover the tooth.
2. If a tooth is avulsed it should be wrapped in a saline-soaked swab and not cleaned. An oral surgeon should be asked for an urgent opinion regarding replantation of any avulsed tooth.

3. If teeth or bridge are damaged an urgent consultation with a dentist must be organized.

4. Dental damage is a frequent cause of litigation. The situation must be explained clearly to the patient and careful records must be made in the case notes.

Nerve damage

When a patient is anaesthetized, protective reflexes are lost and peripheral nerves may be damaged, producing temporary or permanent disability. Nerve damage may not become apparent until up to a week after the injury.

Causes

• Pressure on unprotected nerves such as the facial, common peroneal, or ulnar nerves. This may be due to poor positioning of the patient or direct pressure from equipment, for example a badly applied tourniquet.

• Injection into nerves during induction of anaesthesia, blood gas sampling, or regional anaesthesia.

• Pressure on nerves due to compartment syndrome.

Treatment

1. Prevention is far better than treatment so careful positioning of the patient and gentle techniques during injections are vital.

2. There is no clear evidence that eliciting paraesthesia during local anaesthetic blocks causes nerve damage. However, it would seem logical to limit this to a minimum and perform it gently. Short bevelled needles are less likely to impale nerves, but if they do so they may cause more trauma than long bevelled needles. If a patient complains of severe pain at the start of an injection, suspect intraneural placement and stop injecting.

3. If damage is detected remove the pressure from the area, elevate the limb, and dilute any irritant substances.

4. Provide analgesia.

5. An opinion from a neurologist may be helpful.

Hypersensitivity reactions

Severe reactions occur in about 3 in 10 000 anaesthetics and have a mortality of 4–6 per cent. They are commoner in women. A history of atopy does not increase the risk of an allergic reaction. A previous history of a hypersensitivity should alert the anaesthetist to potential problems. The first sign is often an erythematous rash, but urticaria and periorbital oedema may occur. Cardiac arrhythmias, hypotension, laryngeal oedema (12 per cent of cases), bronchospasm (36–50 per cent of cases), and pulmonary oedema (3 per cent of cases) may develop. In 10 per cent of patients cardiovascular collapse occurs. Patients may develop bleeding and disseminated intravascular coagulation. In 14 per cent of patients the reaction is confined to one system, for example bronchospasm or pulmonary oedema, which may make diagnosis difficult.

Causes

- Drugs. Some drugs are more likely to cause a hypersensitivity reaction, for example antibiotics, thiopentone, suxamethonium, and dextran. Others are less likely to produce reactions, for example etomidate, pancuronium, and vecuronium. Reactions are not always drug specific. Cross-sensitivity can occur between drugs, especially muscle relaxants. A reaction may occur due to overdose, drug incompatibility, or drug interactions.

- Intravenous fluids, hyperosmolar contrast agents, or blood.

- Skin preparations, ethylene oxide, or latex.

Treatment

Anaesthetists should have written protocols for dealing with hypersensitivity reactions. An 'anaphylaxis drill' should be practised regularly.

1. Stop the administration of the agent most likely to be the cause of the reaction, abandon surgery if possible, and call for help.

2. Administer 100 per cent oxygen and intubate earlier rather than later.

3. If cardiac arrest occurs, begin cardiopulmonary resuscitation (see p. 128–131).

4. Pharmacological resuscitation is a priority. Hypotension and broncospasm necessitate administration of adrenaline 100–500 μg intravenously in an adult and 10 μg/kg in a child, which may need to be repeated. Inotrope infusions may be necessary.

5. Treat hypotension with intravenous colloid 10–20 ml/kg. A further reaction to the colloid is unlikely.

6. Consider salbutamol, terbutaline, or aminophylline for adrenaline-resistant bronchospasm. Steroids may be used. Volatile anaesthetics may bronchodilate. Ketamine has been used in this situation.

7. Antihistamine drugs are controversial. H_2 antagonists may be contraindicated.

8. Transfer the patient to a high dependency or intensive care unit as subsequent problems may occur.

9. Discuss the case and send blood samples to a regional immunological centre to determine the cause of the reaction. Measurement of mast cell tryptase is important. Skin tests may be needed, these are usually arranged by the immunology department. Report the reaction to the Committee for Safety of Medicines using the yellow card system.

10. Record the nature of the problem, communicate with the general practitioner, and counsel the patient appropriately.

Further reading

Aitkenhead, A. R. (1990). Awareness during anaesthesia: what should the patient be told. *Anaesthesia*, **45**, 351–2.

Association of Anaesthetists of Great Britain and Ireland (1990). *Anaphylactic reactions with anaesthesia.* A A G B I, London.

Association of Anaesthetists of Great Britain and Ireland and British Society of Allergy and Clinical Immunology (1995). *Suspected anaphylactic reactions associated with anaesthesia.* A A G B I, London

King, T. A. and Adams, A. P. (1990). Failed tracheal intubation. *British Journal of Anaesthesia*, **65**, 400–14.

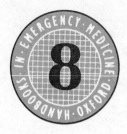

CHAPTER 8

Resuscitation techniques: airway management, ventilation, and defibrillation

Key points in resuscitation techniques: airway management, ventilation, and defibrillation

- It is essential to follow the ABC of resuscitation:
  A clear and maintain the AIRWAY
  B ensure adequate BREATHING
  C ensure adequate CIRCULATION.

- Use 100 per cent oxygen during resuscitation.

- When a cervical spine injury is suspected, use cervical spine control while maintaining the airway. Some patients will need total spinal immobilization.

- In epiglottitis, interference with the airway may cause total airway obstruction.

- All equipment must be ready and checked before intubation is attempted.

- Always have different sizes of tracheal tubes, cut to the correct length.

- Always have a spare working laryngoscope.

- Use a non-cuffed tracheal tube in children aged under 12 years.

- Check the position of the tracheal tube after intubation.
- In a difficult intubation keep the patient well oxygenated and call for help early.
- Oedema of the airway may progress rapidly to total airway obstruction. Patients at risk must be identified early since immediate intubation may be required.
- Careful timing of extubation is essential to avoid complications.
- Emergency cricothyroidotomy is the preferred management of airway obstruction if other methods have failed. Emergency tracheostomy should not be attempted by inexperienced staff.
- Electrical defibrillation is the only effective treatment for established ventricular fibrillation. It is essential to defibrillate as soon as possible.
- Doctors starting a new job should familiarize themselves with the defibrillators used in the hospital. Doctors looking after children should know the correct settings and paddles to use for paediatric resuscitation.
- Some complications of defibrillation can be prevented by attention to technique.
- It is essential that meticulous attention to safety is always given during defibrillation.

Basic and advanced cardiac life support techniques must be second nature to all doctors. These techniques are essential for effective cardiopulmonary resuscitation, and certain individual skills are invaluable when managing patients who are unconscious as a result of trauma, convulsions, poisoning, general anaesthesia, or other causes. Advanced trauma life support (ATLS) techniques are also essential for managing patients with major trauma. Special courses are held to teach these skills.

Basic life support (BLS) techniques should be taught to the general public as well as to all medical, nursing, and paramedical staff. The techniques require no equipment. The Resuscitation Council guidelines for BLS are illustrated in Fig. 8.1 and the European Resuscitation Council guidelines for basic airway management are given in Fig. 8.2. Advanced Life Support (ALS) utilizes medical equipment

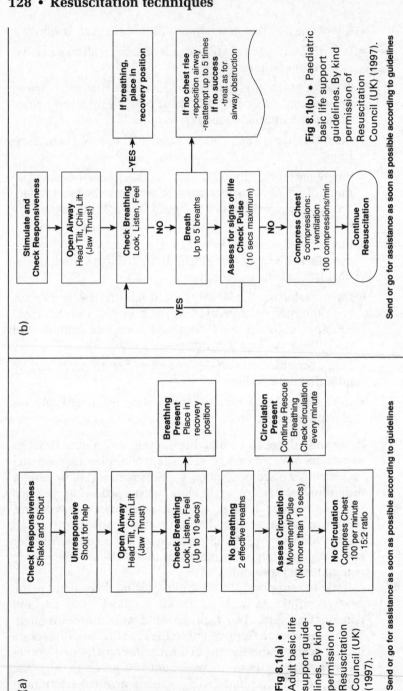

(b)

Stimulate and Check Responsiveness

Open Airway
Head Tilt, Chin Lift
(Jaw Thrust)

Check Breathing
Look, Listen, Feel

— YES → If breathing, place in recovery position

NO

Breath
Up to 5 breaths

→ If no chest rise
- reposition airway
- reattempt up to 5 times
If no success
- treat as for airway obstruction

Assess for signs of life
Check Pulse
(10 secs maximum)

YES

NO

Compress Chest
5 compressions:
1 ventilation
100 compressions/min

Continue Resuscitation

Fig 8.1(b) • Paediatric basic life support guidelines. By kind permission of Resuscitation Council (UK) (1997).

Send or go for assistance as soon as possible according to guidelines

(a)

Check Responsiveness
Shake and Shout

Unresponsive
Shout for help

Open Airway
Head Tilt, Chin Lift
(Jaw Thrust)

Check Breathing
Look, Listen, Feel
(Up to 10 secs)

→ Breathing Present
Place in recovery position

No Breathing
2 effective breaths

Assess Circulation
Movement/Pulse
(No more than 10 secs)

→ Circulation Present
Continue Rescue Breathing
Check circulation every minute

No Circulation
Compress Chest
100 per minute
15:2 ratio

Fig 8.1(a) • Adult basic life support guidelines. By kind permission of Resuscitation Council (UK) (1997).

Send or go for assistance as soon as possible according to guidelines

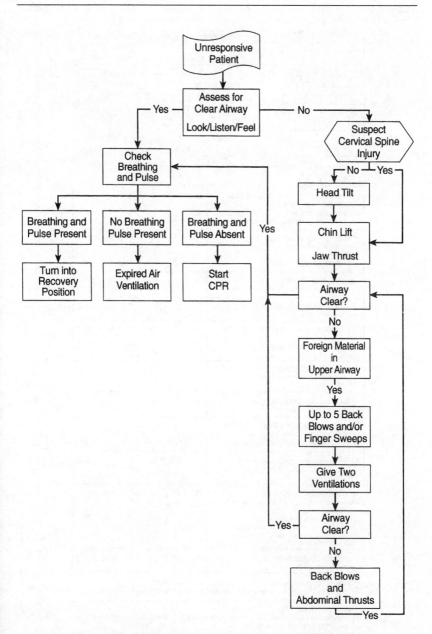

Fig. 8.2 • European Resuscitation Council basic airway management (ERC) guidelines (1996). By kind permission of ERC and Elsevier Science Ireland Ltd.

Table 8.1 • Paediatric resuscitation information. (from Oakley *et al.* 1993)

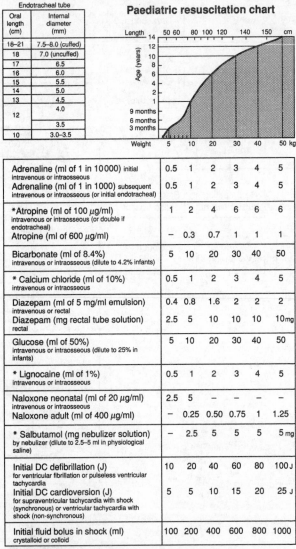

	5	10	20	30	40	50 kg
Adrenaline (ml of 1 in 10000) initial intravenous or intraosseous	0.5	1	2	3	4	5
Adrenaline (ml of 1 in 1000) subsequent intravenous or intraosseous (or initial endotracheal)	0.5	1	2	3	4	5
*Atropine (ml of 100 μg/ml) intravenous or intraosseous (or double if endotracheal)	1	2	4	6	6	6
Atropine (ml of 600 μg/ml)	–	0.3	0.7	1	1	1
Bicarbonate (ml of 8.4%) intravenous or intraosseous (dilute to 4.2% infants)	5	10	20	30	40	50
* Calcium chloride (ml of 10%) intravenous or intraosseous	0.5	1	2	3	4	5
Diazepam (ml of 5 mg/ml emulsion) intravenous or rectal	0.4	0.8	1.6	2	2	2
Diazepam (mg rectal tube solution) rectal	2.5	5	10	10	10	10mg
Glucose (ml of 50%) intravenous or intraosseous (dilute to 25% in infants)	5	10	20	30	40	50
* Lignocaine (ml of 1%) intravenous or intraosseous	0.5	1	2	3	4	5
Naloxone neonatal (ml of 20 μg/ml) intravenous or intraosseous	2.5	5	–	–	–	–
Naloxone adult (ml of 400 μg/ml)	–	0.25	0.50	0.75	1	1.25
* Salbutamol (mg nebulizer solution) by nebulizer (dilute to 2.5–5 ml in physiological saline)	–	2.5	5	5	5	5 mg
Initial DC defibrillation (J) for ventricular fibrillation or pulseless ventricular tachycardia	10	20	40	60	80	100 J
Initial DC cardioversion (J) for supraventricular tachycardia with shock (synchronous) or ventricular tachycardia with shock (non-synchronous)	5	5	10	15	20	25 J
Initial fluid bolus in shock (ml) crystalloid or colloid	100	200	400	600	800	1000

* **Caution!** Non-standard drug concentrations may be available:
Use **atropine** 100 μg/ml or prepare by diluting 1 mg to 10 ml or 600 μg to 6 ml in physiological saline. Note that 1 ml of **calcium chloride** 10% is equivalent to 3 ml of **calcium gluconate** 10%.
Use **lignocaine** (without adrenaline) 1% or give twice the volume of 0.5%: give half the volume of 2% or dilute appropriately.
Salbutamol may also be given by slow intravenous injection (5 μg/kg), but beware the different concentrations available (e.g. 50 and 500 μg/ml).
By kind permission of authors and BMJ Publishing Group.

and drugs. It should be taught to all doctors and to certain groups of nurses and paramedical staff. The Resuscitation Council guidelines for ALS are illustrated in Fig. 8.20 and 8.21. Paediatric resuscitation information is given in Table 8.1.

Airway management: basic life support (BLS) techniques

The aims of airway management are to secure and maintain an adequate airway. Many patients who need resuscitation have an obstructed airway, often as a result of the tongue falling back on the posterior pharyngeal wall. Other common causes of obstruction include vomit and blood. Foreign bodies may occlude the larynx, particularly in children. The airway may be secured by various techniques.

Warning

These techniques involve varying degrees of movement of the cervical spine. Great caution must be exercised in any patient with a suspected neck injury, since inappropriate movement could produce permanent neurological damage. Assume a cervical spine injury in any patient with multi-system trauma, especially with a blunt injury above the clavicle or unconsciousness.

Head tilt

In most cases the tongue can be lifted away from the posterior pharyngeal wall by tilting the head backwards.

Technique
- Tilt the head backwards by placing one hand behind the neck and gently press on the forehead with the other (Fig. 8.3).

Practical points
- Do not over extend the neck in babies and infants, because this may occlude the airway by compressing the larynx against the spine.

- Avoid this technique if a cervical spine injury is suspected.

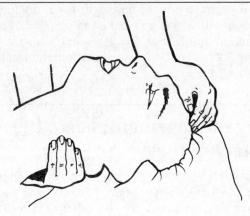

Fig. 8.3 • Head tilt.

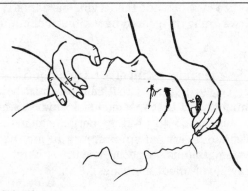

Fig. 8.4 • Chin lift.

Chin lift

The tongue is attached to the mandible, and may be lifted clear by supporting the chin.

Technique
- Place a finger and thumb on top and under the chin and lift it forwards (Fig. 8.4).

Practical points
- Do not push your fingers or thumb under the mandible, since this may compress and occlude the airway, particularly in small children.

- This technique is often used to supplement head tilt; avoid this technique if a cervical spine injury is suspected.

Jaw thrust

This is the most efficient way of opening the airway, but it is not conducive to mouth to mouth ventilation. It is not routinely taught to the general public. This method is used to open the airway while performing bag–valve–mask ventilation.

Technique
- Place the index fingers behind the angle of the mandible and lift this upwards and forwards. The thumbs may be used to depress the point of the chin to open the mouth slightly (Fig. 8.5). Different finger placement is used when holding a mask (see p. 169).

Practical points
- This technique can be performed without moving the neck and is the method of choice when a cervical spine injury is suspected or present.

- Very occasionally this manœuvre may dislocate the jaw.

Recovery position

This may be used:

- For the unconscious or drowsy patient who has a clear, secure airway and adequate spontaneous respiration.

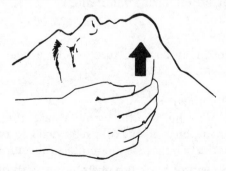

Fig. 8.5 • Jaw thrust.

- To supplement head-down tilt and suction in the unconscious patient who is actively vomiting.

Technique
- Turn the patient into the lateral position and ensure that he cannot roll forwards or backwards.
- Maintain moderate head tilt, with the patient's upper hand placed under the lower cheek.
- Chin lift or jaw thrust should be used where appropriate.

Practical points
- This technique should not be used if the patient has a suspected spinal injury. When it is necessary to turn a patient with a suspected spinal injury 'log-rolling' must be used to ensure that no flexion, extension, or rotational movements are applied to the spine.
- Do not assume that uneventful recovery is guaranteed once the patient is well enough to be placed in the recovery position – careful monitoring is still required to identify any complications.

Clearing the obstructed airway of foreign material

Foreign material occluding the airway may be visible in the mouth. It may be suspected on account of inability to maintain an airway despite careful airway opening or resistance may be felt during ventilation.

Finger sweeps

These may be used to clear the airway of an unconscious patient.

Solid material
- Open the mouth using a jaw thrust technique. The mandible and maxilla may need to be pulled apart posteriorly if there is incomplete relaxation.
- Sweep or hook the obstruction with fingers wrapped in a handkerchief (Fig. 8.6).

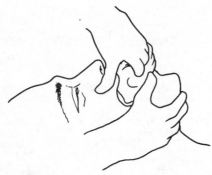

Fig. 8.6 • Finger sweeps.

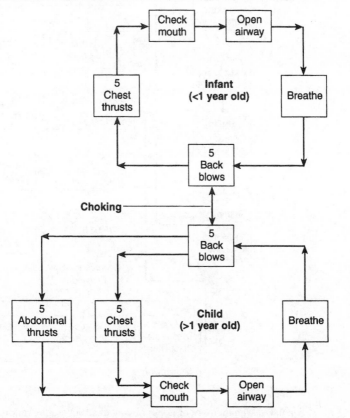

Fig. 8.7 • Management of choking infants and children, from Zideman (1995). By kind permission of author and BMJ Publishing Group.

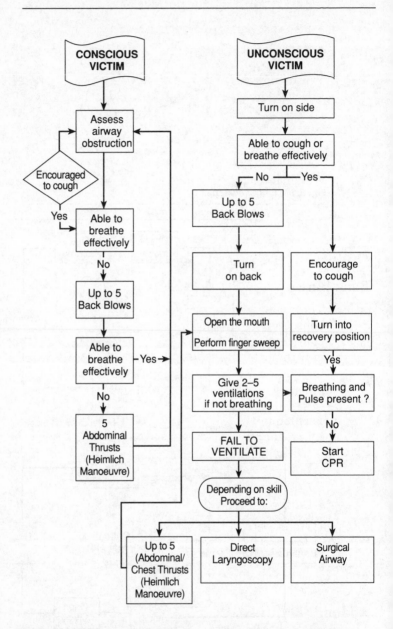

Fig. 8.8 • Management of upper airway obstruction due to foreign material (choking), European Resuscitation Council (ERC) guidelines (1996). By kind permission of ERC and Elsevier Science Ireland Ltd.

Liquid material
- Place the patient head down and turn the head to one side.
- Proceed as before.

Practical points
- Never force the fingers blindly into the back of the throat, since this could cause a sharp foreign body to perforate the pharyngeal wall. It might also stimulate vomiting, gagging, or laryngeal spasm, or might cause the patient to bite the fingers.
- Human bites can cause serious infections therefore always protect your fingers and assess your patient carefully. It is extremely painful to have fingers caught between the clenched teeth of a convulsing patient. It is also very difficult to extricate them.

Back blows

These are used to clear an obstructed upper airway in a conscious patient who cannot relieve the obstruction by coughing. Adults commonly choke on unchewed food and may indicate their dilemma by grasping their neck or pointing to their larynx. Children may choke on unchewed food, pieces of toys, and many other items.

Technique
- Lay the patient on one side. If this is not possible the patient may sit, stand, or lean forward (Fig. 8.9(a)). Children should be placed head down, supported by the rescuer's arm or thigh (Fig. 8.9(b,c)).
- During expiration give five blows in the middle of the back, between the shoulder blades.

Practical point
- This technique may be used in unconscious patients.

Abdominal thrusts

The conscious patient – the Heimlich manœuvre
This may be used to expel an impacted foreign body from a conscious patient if back blows have been unsuccessful.

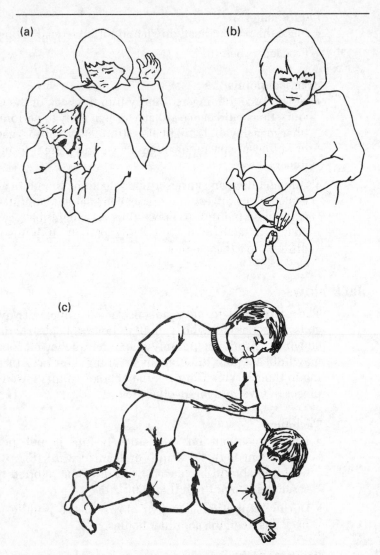

Fig. 8.9 • Back blow: (a) adult, (b) baby, (c) child.

- Stand behind the patient and place the arms around the patient just below the rib cage.
- Clasp the hands firmly together over the epigastrium and give a series of upward thrusts in time with expiration (Fig. 8.10).

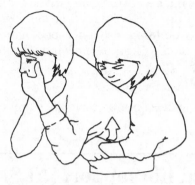

Fig. 8.10 • Heimlich manœuvre.

- If this fails the patient may lose consciousness and must then be laid down; attempts may then be made to remove the obstruction by finger sweeps.

The unconscious patient
- Lay the patient supine and kneel at the side of the abdomen (small rescuers may find it easier to kneel astride the patient).
- Place the heel of one hand on the epigastrium and the heel of the other hand on the dorsum of the carpus.
- Give a series of upward thrusts; then clear the airway with finger sweeps.
- If this fails continue basic life support and try back blows.

Practical point
- Abdominal thrusts may cause visceral injury to stomach, spleen, liver, aorta, and diaphragm. It is not recommended for children, during pregnancy, or for extreme obesity.

Chest compression – the unconscious patient

This technique may be used to dislodge impacted foreign bodies in the unconscious patient who is a child, pregnant, or obese.

Technique
- Lay the patient supine and kneel at the side of the chest.

- Place the heel of one hand in the centre of the sternum and place the heel of the other hand on top. In infants and small children use only one hand; use the forefinger and middle finger of one hand for babies.
- Give a series of chest compressions; then clear the airway with finger sweeps.
- If this fails continue basic life support and try back blows.

Advanced life support (ALS) techniques

If the airway cannot be maintained using BLS techniques then ALS measures using equipment should be employed as soon as possible.

Foreign material removal

Foreign material may be removed from the upper airway of an unconscious patient under direct vision using a laryngoscope, suction, and Magill forceps.

Technique
- Open the airway by head tilt.
- Introduce the laryngoscope blade into the right side of the mouth and direct the blade towards the midline at laryngeal level.
- Lift the laryngoscope blade upwards and forwards – this lifts the tongue clear of the posterior pharyngeal wall and provides direct vision of the pharynx.
- Use a Yankauer-type suction catheter to remove liquid and small solids.
- Larger solid material can be picked out with Magill forceps (Fig. 8.11).

Practical points
- Do not lever on the upper incisors with the laryngoscope, as this may damage the teeth and obscure the view of the hypopharynx.
- Use the suction gently: rough use may cause trauma and haemorrhage.

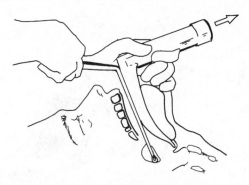

Fig. 8.11 • Foreign body removal with Magill forceps.

Oropharyngeal (Guedel) airway

This is used in the unconscious patient to hold the tongue away from the posterior pharyngeal wall. Basic techniques of opening the airway may still be needed to maintain a patent airway.

Insertion of an oropharyngeal airway

- Select the appropriate size of airway by placing the airway against the patient's face. The correctly sized airway will extend from the centre of the mouth to the angle of the jaw.

- Have airways of one size larger and one size smaller ready (see Table 3.4, p. 53).

- Insert the airway, with its concave side towards the hard palate to avoid pushing the tongue backwards into the throat. With the tip near the pharyngeal end of the hard palate rotate the airway while inserting it, until the bite-block is between the teeth. The flange should lie on but not inside the lips, and the concave side will be against the tongue (Fig. 8.12).

- In a small child, airway insertion should be aided using a tongue depressor or laryngoscope blade. The airway is inserted with the concave surface facing downwards. The airway should not be rotated in the mouth due to the risk of trauma.

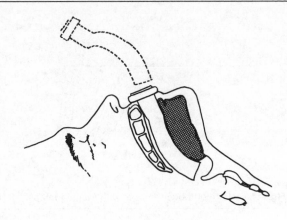

Fig. 8.12 • Insertion of oropharyngeal airway.

Contraindications
- **Never** insert an oropharyngeal airway if epiglottitis is suspected, as total airway obstruction may be precipitated.

Complications
- Damage to teeth or soft tissues of the mouth may occur, particularly if attempts are made to force the airway between clenched teeth.
- Gagging, vomiting, aspiration, or laryngospasm may arise in patients with active laryngeal reflexes, particularly if too large an airway is used. Remove the airway if these occur.
- Too small an airway will not hold the tongue clear of the pharyngeal wall and the end of the airway may be occluded by the tongue.

Practical points
- A small oral airway is often useful in the edentulous elderly patient whose face seems to 'cave in' in the absence of teeth.
- An oral airway may help stabilize an oral tracheal tube during transfer of the patient. It can be placed at the side of the tube, but is no substitute for careful securing of the tube.

- A patient may bite on a tracheal tube, thus occluding the airway. A small oral airway placed carefully at the side of the tracheal tube may protect the latter while control is regained.
- A patient who spits the airway out usually does not need one.
- Oral airways may be difficult to insert if the patient is clenching his or her teeth. Never try to force an airway in. It is better to try a nasopharyngeal airway.

Nasopharyngeal airway

This may be used in either nostril to provide a patent airway between the nostril and the laryngeal opening (Fig 8.13).

Insertion of a nasopharyngeal airway
- Select the appropriate size of airway. The diameter of the airway should be approximately equal to the diameter of the patient's little finger.
- Have airways of one size larger and one size smaller ready.
- Choose the nostril which appears the most patent. Septal deviation causes narrowing of a nostril.
- Lubricate the tube with water soluble jelly.
- Guide the airway through the nostril. If an obstruction prevents passage of the airway try the other nostril.
- Attempts to force the airway down will cause trauma and bleeding.
- The flange should lie against but not inside the nostril.
- Always have suction at hand to control any nasal bleeding.

Contraindications
- **Never** insert a nasopharyngeal airway if epiglottitis is suspected, as total airway obstruction may be precipitated.
- A nasopharyngeal airway is best avoided in patients with a bleeding diathesis.
- Do not use a nasopharyngeal airway in patients with a suspected basal skull or facial fracture.

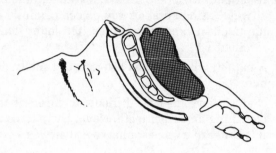

Fig. 8.13 • Insertion of nasopharyngeal airway.

Practical points

- Nasopharyngeal airways are generally better tolerated than oropharyngeal ones. They are particularly useful where insertion of an oral airway is difficult, for example, in cases of trismus or decerebrate rigidity, or when the patient is fitting.

- A suction catheter may be introduced via a nasopharyngeal airway to facilitate pharyngeal suction. Always ensure that the airway is patent after this procedure.

Tracheal intubation

Tracheal intubation is used to provide a secure, clear airway, through which positive pressure ventilation may be applied. Gastric inflation and aspiration of gastric contents are prevented once the tube is correctly sited with its cuff inflated. Orotracheal intubation is the most commonly used method. The nastotracheal route is less commonly used. It requires more skill and in resuscitation situations is usually reserved for occasions when orotracheal intubation is impossible. It may also be preferentially used with confirmed cervical spine injuries. The nasotracheal tube can be introduced blindly or under direct vision. Blind intubation may be used in the spontaneously breathing patient by experienced operators. Certain drugs may be given down the tracheal tube during the management of a cardiac arrest. Tracheal intubation requires considerable practice and skill. Any doctor likely to require this skill must at a minimum receive training on a manikin.

Indications
- Any cardiorespiratory arrest lasting more than 2–3 minutes
- To secure a patent airway
- To prevent aspiration
- To control or correct ventilation
- To administer drugs
- For anaesthesia
- To facilitate tracheo-bronchial toilet

Contraindications
- **Never** attempt laryngoscopy or tracheal intubation in a spontaneously breathing patient suspected of having epiglottitis. This may convert a partial into a total airway obstruction. Tracheal intubation may be the treatment of choice but this must be performed by a senior anaesthetist using controlled anaesthesia.
- Special caution: If tracheal intubation is required in a patient with a suspected cervical spine injury midline immobilization of the head and neck is mandatory.

Equipment
- Suction (Yankauer and bronchial catheters)
- Laryngoscope and a spare, with interchangeable blades of appropriate sizes
- Selection of oral and nasal tracheal tubes of different diameters and cut to the appropriate lengths (An average size adult male will need a 9.0 and a female will need an 8.0) (p. 56)
- Suitable connection to ventilation apparatus
- 10 ml syringe to inflate the cuff
- Flexible stylet
- Gum-elastic bougie
- Lubricating water soluble jelly
- Magill forceps
- Tape to secure the tube
- Throat pack for children

Before attempting intubation always check that:

- the suction and the laryngoscopes are working
- the cuffs on the tracheal tubes do not leak
- the syringe is full of air
- the tracheal tube, connector, and ventilating device all connect together correctly.

Ideally an assistant should perform cricoid pressure, inflate the cuff, and pass equipment as necessary.

Orotracheal intubation

- Place the patient in the supine position with a pillow under the head.
- Extend the head on the neck by placing a hand on the forehead and pushing the occiput caudally. This manœuvre is appropriate only in patients with no cervical spine trauma.
- Hold the laryngoscope in the left hand with the tip of the blade pointing towards the ceiling.
- Insert the laryngoscope into the right side of the mouth, using the right fingers to keep the lips free from the laryngoscope blade.
- Advance the laryngoscope blade towards the midline. Always keep the tongue to the left of the blade.
- Lift the laryngoscope, handle forwards and upwards, away from the face (Fig. 8.14). Adjust the tip of a curved blade so that it lies between the base of the tongue and the root of the epiglottis (Fig. 8.15a). The tip of a straight blade should lie beneath the epiglottis (Fig. 8.15b).
- Visualize the vocal cords, adjusting the blade if necessary to get the best view. Cricoid pressure may help bring the vocal cords into view.
- Insert the tracheal tube into the right side of the mouth. Guide it along the length of the laryngoscope blade and pass it between the vocal cords under direct vision. The cuff must lie below the vocal cords.
- Attach the tube to a self-inflating bag or anaesthetic circuit, making sure that their weight does not dislodge the tube.

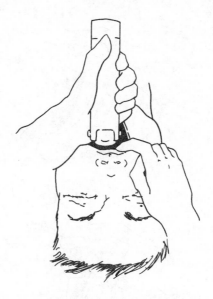

Fig. 8.15 • Insertion of laryngoscope.

- Inflate the cuff with air through the pilot tube while ventilating the patient. Use just enough air to prevent a leak occurring around the tube.
- Check that the tube is correctly placed by observing chest-wall movement and listening for breath sounds over the upper and lower lobes of both lungs, and over the stomach.
- Secure the tube firmly in place.

Practical points
- Ensure adequate ventilation and oxygenation before intubation is attempted. Take a deep breath as you start intubation. The patient should be intubated before you have to breathe again. If this time is exceeded without successful intubation remove the laryngoscope and tube and ventilate the patient with 100 per cent oxygen via a bag and mask for 1–2 minutes before repeating the procedure.

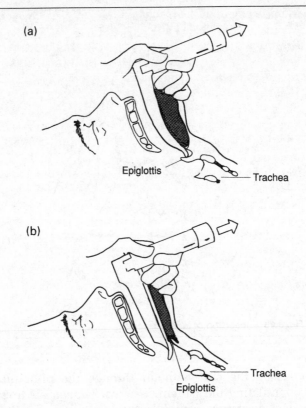

Fig. 8.15 • Position of (a) curved and (b) straight laryngoscope blade and epiglottis.

- Intubation is facilitated by muscle relaxation, which may be a result of coma or deliberately induced as part of an anaesthetic technique. Intubation should not be attempted in patients with sufficient muscle tone to bite on the laryngoscope blade, gag, or cough, since it may result in trauma to the mouth or pharynx, laryngeal spasm, or vomiting and aspiration. Intubation may cause increases in intracranial and intraocular pressures.
- The tip of the tracheal tube should be in the middle third of the trachea with the head in the neutral position. Flexion of the head advances the tracheal tube by a mean of 1.9 cm and extension of the head withdraws the tube by a mean of 1.9 cm.

Misplacement of the tracheal tube

Misplacement of the tracheal tube in the oesophagus is a common problem that may cause hypoxaemia and death if left undiagnosed. Oesophageal intubation is more likely to occur with inexperience and during a difficult intubation. However, anyone who fails to think about the problem may miss it. Clinical signs can prove unreliable. Gas passing through the oesophagus may mimic normal breath sounds and chest movement. A 'bubbling' sound over the stomach may not always be heard when ventilating the oesophagus but the latter may produce good chest wall movement, as well as abdominal distension. Correct placement can be confirmed by measuring end-tidal carbon dioxide for at least five ventilatory cycles, demonstrating the movement of the bag when spontaneous ventilation restarts, or performing a chest radiograph. However, these signs are not applicable in many situations. The patient's response to intubation may be a good indication of the tube position. The tube is likely to be in place if a blue patient becomes pink but if a pink patient goes blue it is probably not. These possibilities require some cardiovascular output. Direct vision of the tube passing through the cords confirms its initial correct placement but the tube may subsequently slip into the pharynx.

The oesophageal detector device has been designed to aid diagnosis of misplacement of the tracheal tube, and relies upon the relative rigidity of the trachea compared with the oesophagus (Williams and Nunn 1989). The oesophagus collapses over the end of a rigid tube when a negative pressure is applied to it, thus preventing aspiration of air. Free aspiration of air from the trachea can occur in such circumstances, because the wall does not collapse. An Ellick's evacuator bulb is attached to a tracheal tube connector, which is connected to the tracheal tube. Squeezing the bulb produces a characteristic flatus-like noise if the tube is in the oesophagus. Release of the bulb is followed by absent or markedly delayed filling. With the tube in the trachea emptying the bulb is silent, and refill is instantaneous.

If oesophageal intubation has occurred the tube should be removed immediately and the patient should be ventilated with oxygen before any further attempts at intubation are made. The aphorism 'if in doubt take it out' still holds true if misplacement of the tube is suspected.

The tracheal tube may also be misplaced into the right main bronchus, resulting in collapse of the left lung or pneumothorax. This may occur if too long a tube is used, particularly in children. Observation of chest movement and auscultation of both upper lobes of the lungs should help identify this problem, which is rectified by slowly withdrawing the tube until both lungs are ventilated equally.

Complications of intubation
- Inability to intubate due to:
  (a) inadequate training or experience
  (b) inadequate equipment
  (c) inadequate relaxation
  (d) facial deformity (trauma, poorly developed mandible, anteriorly placed larynx)
  (e) airway obstruction (trauma, oedema, haemorrhage)
- Induction of vomiting
- Oesophageal intubation
- Right main bronchus intubation
- Tracheal tube
  (a) rupture and leak from the cuff
  (b) size incorrect, predisposing to misplacement or leak around tube
- Mouth and airway
  (a) chipping or loosening of teeth (caused by levering with laryngoscope)
  (b) haemorrhage secondary to trauma
  (c) dislocation of mandible
  (d) trauma to vocal cords (particularly if too large a tube is used)
- Damage to cervical spine and/or spinal cord
- Sore throat following traumatic intubation

Nasotracheal intubation
- Place the patient in the supine position with a pillow under the head.
- Extend the head on the neck by placing a hand on the forehead and pushing the occiput caudally.

- Lubricate the nasotracheal tube and introduce it into a nostril.
- Guide the tube gently but firmly along the nasal passage, to avoid the large inferior turbinate. If the tube will not pass along the nostril remove the tube and try the other side.
- Continue to guide the tube as it passes downwards through the pharynx to the larynx.
- Insert the tube under direct vision. Visualize the glottis using a laryngoscope, and with the right hand hold the tube from its distal end with Magill forceps. Steer the tube through the glottis while the assistant gently pushes the tube at the nasal end (Fig. 8.17).
- If the tube passes between the cords but then impacts anteriorly, it may be dislodged by rotating the tube through 90° or slightly flexing the head on the neck.
- Inflate the cuff and check that the tube is in the correct place.
- Secure the tube.

Practical points
- A vasoconstrictor such as oxymetazoline may be used in the nostril to reduce the risk of haemorrhage. However, this may take up to 20 minutes to be fully effective, and is thus not appropriate for use in emergency situations.

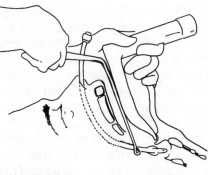

Fig. 8.16 • Nasal intubation.

- Blind nasotracheal intubation can be used in the spontaneously breathing conscious patient. The airway should first be anaesthetized with local anaesthetic (see p. 376). Listen for breath sounds as the tube is guided to the larynx. This will aid correct placement of the tube.

- Avoid holding the tube cuff in the Magill forceps, as these may puncture it. The cuff may sometimes be punctured by sharp turbinate bones. If the cuff is punctured and leaking the tube must be replaced.

- Prolonged attempts at intubation may cause hypoxaemia. Always ensure that the patient is adequately oxygenated.

Complications

These are similar to those for orotracheal intubation, with the added complication of trauma to the nasal passages and nasopharynx and brisk bleeding. Submucosal passage of the tube may occur; if so, remove the tube, and be alert for subsequent infection. Nasotracheal intubation is contra-indicated in patients with facial or base of skull fracture.

Tracheal intubation in infants and small children

The technique is essentially the same for children as for adults but there are some important differences. The infant's larynx is higher in the neck than the adult and may be more difficult to visualize. The epiglottis is relatively large and floppy. It is therefore best to use a straight-bladed laryngoscope for infants up to the age of about 6 months. The narrowest part of the glottis in an adult is between the vocal cords but in a child it is at the cricoid ring. A tube may thus pass easily through the cords, only to get stuck just below. Never force a tube past the cricoid ring, as it may cause trauma, resulting in postoperative stridor and subsequent stenosis. If the tube will not pass through the cricoid ring always change to a tube one size smaller. Trauma at the cricoid level can also be reduced by using non-cuffed tubes, which should always be used in children aged 12 years or under. A slight leak should be apparent after intubation of a child if the tube size is correct. The trachea in a child is relatively short, so it is easy to intubate the bronchus. Always check the position of the tube carefully. The tube may be secured by a moistened throat pack, in addition to tape.

Choice of tube size

Correct choice of tube size is essential to minimize the risk of trauma to the larynx. If the tube size is correct there should just be a small gas leak around it. Excessive gas leakage around the tube may occur when the diameter is too small; or the tube may be misplaced into the right main bronchus if the tube is too long. Always have available tubes one size larger and one one size smaller than the anticipated size (see Table 3.6, p. 56). Never force a tube between or below the cords, but try a size smaller. If in adults there is a leak around the tube despite the cuffs being inflated with 10–15 ml air, use a larger tube. Tube sizes for children may be calculated from the following formulae:

$$\text{Internal diameter (mm)} = \frac{\text{age in years}}{4} + 4.0$$

$$\text{Length of orotracheal tube (cm)} = \frac{\text{age in years}}{2} + 12.0$$

$$\text{Length of nasotracheal tube (cm)} = \frac{\text{age in years}}{2} + 15.0$$

Tracheal intubation and cervical spine injuries

Movement of the neck may cause spinal cord damage in a patient with an unstable injury of the cervical spine. In trauma patients, 25 per cent of cervical spine injuries may be caused by improper handling during prehospital care. Every patient with multiple trauma should be presumed to have a neck injury, especially if there is blunt trauma above the clavicle. Any patient with a head and chest injury should be presumed to have a cervical spine injury. A lateral cervical spine radiograph including the C7/T1 interspace may demonstrate an unstable injury, but cannot conclusively exclude one. In all suspected and confirmed cases of cervical spine injury the neck should be immobilized, either by manual in-line immobilization or with a correctly sized hard collar, sand bags, and adhesive tape across the forehead and chin attached to either side of the trolley. The airway should be maintained by a jaw-thrust technique, with an oral or nasal airway where appropriate. Tracheal intubation should be performed with midline manual immobilization of the head and neck by a trained assistant. The use of a rigid collar alone increases the difficulty of intubation because it reduces mouth opening. It does not contribute to neck stability during laryngoscopy. If there is time, call for the help of an experienced anaesthetist in this situation.

Cricoid pressure (Sellick's manœuvre)

This manœuvre aims to prevent regurgitation by occluding the oesophagus between the cricoid cartilage and the vertebral column. The tips of the thumb and first two fingers of one hand are placed either side of the cricoid cartilage and backward pressure is applied when directed by the anaesthetist (Fig. 8.17). The pressure is applied just before induction of anaesthesia, or as the patient loses consciousness. It is best to warn the patient that some pressure may be felt on the neck as he or she goes off to sleep. The pressure should not be released until the tracheal tube cuff is inflated and the airway has been secured. Cricoid pressure should not be used during active vomiting as oesophageal rupture may occur. Badly applied cricoid pressure may increase the difficulty of intubation.

Difficult intubation

All anaesthetists will face this problem at some time and it is important to have a clear plan of action for when it occurs.

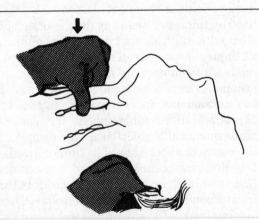

Figure 8.17 • Cricoid pressure.

The skill in managing a difficult intubation is to anticipate the problem and call for expert help sooner rather than later. It is also vital to remember that no matter what happens the patient must be kept well oxygenated. This can often be done using well practised basic and advanced life-support techniques.

Common causes of difficult airway control and intubation

Inexperience

The inexperienced doctor often creates problems for himself by not following the basic rules of airway management. A difficult intubation suddenly becomes possible with attention to detail. Common faults include failure to check the equipment, poor positioning of the patient, forgetting to ventilate the patient with oxygen before and between attempts, taking too long over each attempt, and not calling for help soon enough. Confusion sometimes arises between the optimal head position for airway opening during mouth to mouth ventilation compared with that for tracheal intubation. The former is often easier without a pillow under the head. For tracheal intubation it is vital to start with a pillow under the head and, if the vocal cords cannot be seen, to double the pillow up. Too often inexperienced doctors remove the pillow but this often only makes things worse.

Situation

Difficult intubations are often easier to perform in the operating theatre, where trained assistance and familiar equipment are available. It is often impossible to transfer emergency patients immediately from the resuscitation room. The A & E department must therefore have adequate resuscitation equipment to manage the common emergencies.

Equipment

Intubation equipment may fail in an emergency, be borrowed and not returned, or be replaced by a new piece of equipment incompatible with the rest of the system. It is vital to check all the equipment before attempting intubation.

Trauma

Face

Facial fractures with associated haemorrhage and swelling distort the normal anatomy and obstruct the airway. There is an increased risk of vomiting and aspiration from swallowed blood. Head-down tilt may aid clearing of the airway with suction. Some patients need to be face down to maintain a patent airway. Facial fractures may be unstable but do not usually cause problems in visualizing the cords. The major problem comes from swelling and haemorrhage and may necessitate intubation. The patient may be conscious despite severe facial injuries and anaesthesia is required for intubation. This must be performed by an experienced anaesthetist.

Neck

Soft tissue swelling and haemorrhage may necessitate early intubation. Cervical spine injuries complicate intubation, because the head and neck must be immobilized (see p. 153). If the larynx is difficult to visualize, ask an assistant to push the larynx posteriorly. If there is no improvement try moving the larynx laterally in case it has been displaced from the midline. Consider using a different laryngoscope blade, try a larger blade, or perhaps change to a straight one or a McCoy blade. It may be easier to direct the tube to the larynx using a stylet or gum elastic bougie. If the tube will not go past the vocal cords, try a smaller tube. Nasotracheal intubation should be considered as long as there is no base of skull fracture.

Larynx

Fracture of the larynx may require an emergency surgical airway (see p. 161).

Anatomical variations

An experienced anaesthetist can quickly identify the types of head and neck which cause problems during intubation (Fig. 8.18). The most obvious are gross facial deformities,

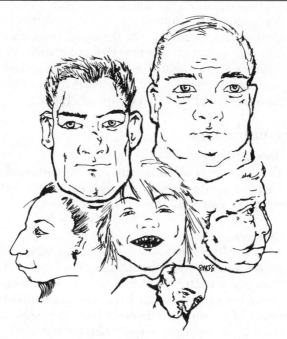

Fig. 8.18 • The many faces of a difficult intubation.

such as the Treacher–Collins syndrome. Large faces associated with acromegaly may also cause problems. Less obvious but equally difficult are those patients with a poorly developed mandible that reduces the space available for the tongue in the oropharynx. The patient with a short distance between the hyoid and the mandible may also be difficult to intubate. Gross dental deformity presents problems, especially when associated with loose teeth. Difficulties may also arise with obese, bull-necked, or arthritic patients, and with those with ankylosing spondylitis. The non-anaesthetist should be able to identify many of these conditions, or to suspect their presence if there has been a problem in maintaining the airway.

Oropharyngeal airways may help to maintain the airway but should not be used if the dentition is very poor. Nasopharyngeal airways are particularly useful if the problem is at the level of the tongue. In the extreme situation it may be necessary to pull the tongue forward, using a tongue-clip placed in the dorsum of the tongue. This not only pulls the tongue away from the posterior pharyngeal wall but also elevates the epiglottis. The laryngeal mask may provide the best airway but its use requires experience. Ventilating the difficult airway with the bag–valve–mask technique often requires two people, one to hold the mask in place and open the airway, and the other to squeeze the bag.

Airway obstruction

Haemorrhage
This may be controlled with suction and head-down tilt. It often necessitates early intubation and in extreme cases, emergency surgical airway.

Oedema
Airway oedema can develop with alarming speed and may cause total airway obstruction, hypoxia, and death. The emergency doctor must identify those patients at risk and obtain expert anaesthetic help. The treatment of oedema as a result of anaphylaxis is described on p. 124. Intubation of infants and children with obstruction due to infection should be performed by an experienced anaesthetist. Never disturb the airway of a patient with airway obstruction who is breathing spontaneously, since this may result in complete obstruction. Burns involving the airway can be disastrous because of sudden airway obstruction. Children who have inhaled steam from a kettle or teapot are also at particular risk of airway obstruction. There may initially be no obvious sign of oedema or airway obstruction. The emergency doctor must always look for indications of inhalation injury, since the correct management of this consists of immediate tracheal intubation before the airway becomes obstructed and difficult to intubate. The signs of inhalation injury are:

- a hoarse voice
- stridor
- facial burns
- singeing of the eyebrows and nasal hair
- carbon deposits and acute inflammatory changes in the oropharynx

- carbonaceous sputum and
- a history of an impaired mental state and/or being confined in a burning environment.

Foreign body

A foreign body causing obstruction can often be suspected from the history and must always be considered in small children with airway problems. The removal of foreign bodies is described on p. 134. Occasionally an emergency surgical airway is required. Rigid bronchoscopy may be needed to remove foreign bodies from the airway.

Inadequate relaxation

Non-anaesthetists sometimes cause problems by attempting to intubate a patient who has some voluntary muscle tone and laryngeal reflexes. The patient will then not tolerate the laryngoscope in the mouth, let alone intubation. Orotracheal intubation requires good muscle relaxation. This may require the use of anaesthesia and muscle relaxants, thus an anaesthetist must be called. Adequate anaesthesia is essential for intubation of head injured patients, otherwise the intracranial pressure may increase dramatically.

Failed intubation

This is discussed on p. 107.

Extubation

A patient should not be extubated until he or she is breathing spontaneously and has regained active laryngeal reflexes. Premature extubation may cause hypoxaemia due to hypoventilation, apnoea or airway obstruction. Regurgitation and aspiration may occur. A delay in extubation may result in laryngeal trauma due to the patient coughing or pulling on the tube. The patient may also develop laryngeal spasm if the depth of anaesthesia is incorrect during extubation.

Equipment

The patient should be on a trolley which allows head-down tilt. Suction should be working and all the equipment and drugs necessary for re-intubation must be immediately available. An oxygen supply, oxygen mask, and oropharyngeal airways are also required.

Technique

- Have an assistant available, since it is difficult to deal with complications single-handed.
- Patients sometimes have to lie supine but if possible the patient should lie on his left side, particularly when regurgitation or vomiting may be expected.
- Gently use suction to clear any saliva from the mouth under direct vision.
- Untie the tape securing the tube but ensure that the tube does not fall out prematurely.
- Deflate the cuff when spontaneous respiration returns but before the patient coughs on the tube.
- Remove the tube once the laryngeal reflexes are present.
- Check that the airway is patent and that ventilation is adequate. An oropharyngeal airway is sometimes needed at this stage.
- Give the patient oxygen by face mask.

Complications

- Trauma to larynx, pharynx, or mouth
- Hypoventilation
- Laryngeal spasm
- Vomiting and aspiration

Tracheal administration of drugs

Atropine and lignocaine may be given via the tracheal tube when managing a cardiac arrest. Adrenaline can also be given this way, but vasoconstriction may reduce its absorption. Twice the intravenous dose should be given. The drugs may take longer to have an effect than if given intravenously. This route can be used if there is delay in obtaining venous access. **Never** give sodium bicarbonate or calcium solutions into the trachea.

Emergency cricothyroidotomy

This may take the form of needle or surgical cricothyroidotomy. The former is used in children under 12 years of age. Emergency tracheostomy is not advisable. It is difficult to perform, it may take a long time to complete, and it can also produce bleeding.

Indication

Inability to intubate the trachea is the only indication for creating a surgical airway during resuscitation. This may occur in situations such as severe oropharyngeal haemorrhage, oedema of the glottis, fracture of the larynx, or foreign body obstruction at the larynx.

Needle cricothyroidotomy with jet insufflation of the airway

Technique
- Place the patient in the supine position (Fig. 8.19). Extend the head and place a pillow or sandbag under the shoulders if there is no cervical spine injury.
- Locate the cricothyroid membrane between the thyroid and cricoid cartilages.
- Clean the overlying skin with antiseptic.
- Attach a 12 gauge intravenous cannula to a 5 or 10 ml syringe.
- Puncture the skin in the midline over the cricothyroid membrane; then direct the needle caudally at an angle of 45°.
- Insert the needle through the lower half of the cricothyroid membrane, aspirating as the needle is advanced.

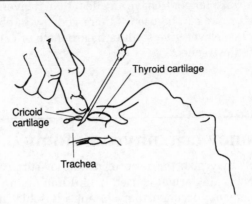

Cricoid cartilage

Thyroid cartilage

Trachea

Fig. 8.19 • Emergency needle cricothyroidotomy.

- Aspiration of air indicates entry into the trachea.
- Advance the cannula downward into the trachea while withdrawing the needle.
- At all times ensure that the cannula is not dislodged.
- Attach the cannula to previously prepared oxygen tubing. This should have a Y connector or be cut with a side hole and is prepared from oxygen tubing with an adaptable male–female link. One connector is trimmed so that it will fit securely over the end of the cannula. The other end should fit over an oxygen supply portal. A hole 3.0 mm in diameter is cut about 6.0 cm from the patient end of the tubing.
- Use an oxygen flow rate of 15 litres/min. (345 kPa). Intermittently ventilate the lungs by covering the hole in the tubing with a finger at a rate of one second on to four seconds off.
- Assess the patient's oxygenation.
- Secure the cannula to the patient's neck.

Practical points
- Some exhalation occurs during the four seconds that oxygen is not being delivered under pressure. Carbon dioxide retention gradually occurs because of inadequate ventilation, and thus the technique is only suitable for 30 to 45 minutes.

- A second cannula may be inserted through the crico-thyroid membrane if there is insufficient airway for exhalation either through the cannula or the larynx.
- The high pressure gas flow may be sufficient to expel into the hypopharynx a foreign body impacted in the larynx.

Complications
- Asphyxia
- Haemorrhage
- Posterior tracheal wall perforation
- Oesophageal perforation
- Thyroid perforation
- Subcutaneous and/or mediastinal emphysema
- Haematoma formation
- Aspiration
- Cellulitis
- Inadequate ventilation, causing hypercapnia and hypox-aemia.

Surgical cricothyroidotomy

Technique
- Place the patient in the supine position (Fig. 8.21). Extend the head and place a pillow under the shoulders if there is no cervical spine injury.
- Locate the cricothyroid membrane between the thyroid and cricoid cartilages.
- Clean the overlying skin with antiseptic and anaesthetize the site of incision with local anaesthetic with adrenaline.
- Make a 2–3 cm horizontal midline incision over the lower half of the cricothyroid membrane.
- Identify and incise the membrane sufficient to insert a 5–7 mm tube.
- The opening may be dilated using a curved haemostat or by inserting the scalpel handle and rotating it through 90°.
- Insert a tube of the appropriate size into the trachea, under direct vision, directing it distally. A cuffed tracheostomy tube is preferable but a cuffed tracheal tube may be used.

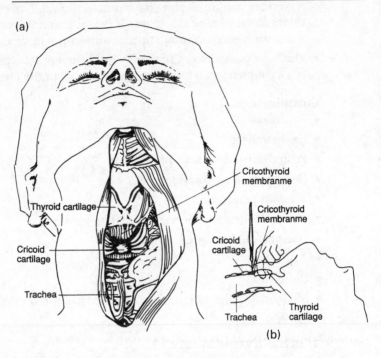

(a)

Cricothyroid membranme

Thyroid cartilage

Cricoid cartilage

Trachea

Cricothyroid membranme

Cricoid cartilage

Trachea

Thyroid cartilage

(b)

Fig. 8.20 • Emergency surgical cricothyroidotomy: (a) and (b) frontal and lateral views.

- Inflate the cuff and ventilate the patient.
- Assess the patient for adequate ventilation and oxygenation.
- Secure the tube to the patient's neck.

Practical points
- Never cut or remove the cricoid cartilage. The cricoid cartilage is the only circumferential support to the trachea in children. Surgical cricothyroidotomy is not recommended in children under 12 years of age.
- Ensure the opening is large enough to accommodate the tube, otherwise the tube may take the line of least resistance and pass pretracheally. Forcing the tube into the trachea must be avoided, since this may cause major complications.

- Cricothyroidotomy sets are available. These are used in intensive care units to facilitate bronchial toilet. They use a 'blind technique', and some use only plain tubes. It is better to use a 'direct vision' technique and cuffed tube in an emergency.

Complications
- Asphyxia
- Haemorrhage
- Creation of a false passage into the tissues
- Laceration of the trachea
- Laceration of the oesophagus
- Mediastinal emphysema
- Aspiration
- Cellulitis
- Haematoma formation
- Laryngeal stenosis
- Subglottic stenosis/oedema
- Vocal cord paralysis, hoarseness

Ventilation: basic life support (BLS) techniques

Mouth to mouth ventilation

This technique should be used to ventilate an apnoeic patient unless equipment is immediately to hand.

Technique
- Lay the patient supine and open the airway. Work from the side of the patient.
- Squeeze the nose to close the nostrils.
- Support the chin with the other hand and hold the mouth about 2 cm open.
- Take a deep breath and seal your mouth around that of the patient.
- Blow into the patient's mouth until the chest rises.

- At the end of inhalation remove your mouth to allow passive expiration of the patient. The technique can then be repeated.

Practical points
- If a cervical spine injury is suspected extend the head as little as is necessary to open the airway.
- Cross infection with viral or bacterial infections could occur during mouth to mouth ventilation. Consider antibiotic prophylaxis for those potentially in contact with bacterial infections.
- A face shield may be used to reduce the risk of infection transmission during mouth to mouth (or mouth to nose) ventilation. This consists of a filter welded on to a plastic sheet. The filter is placed across the patient's nose and mouth. The filter repels fluid and reduces the passage of aerosol-borne micro organisms. The filter has a low resistance.
- Difficulty with inflation may occur with poor airway position. Extend the head tilt, or try chin lift and jaw thrust techniques. A poorly opened airway will encourage ventilation of the stomach. A distended stomach will 'splint' the diaphragm and further impede ventilation. There will also be an increased risk of regurgitation and aspiration. Foreign material may obstruct the airway and should be cleared with finger sweeps, back blows, or abdominal thrusts (see p. 136). Inadequate occlusion of the nose may allow an air leak and thus reduce inflation efficiency.

Mouth to nose ventilation

This method is useful in cases of trismus or mandibular injury, or where there are cultural objections to the mouth to mouth technique.

Technique
- Position the patient as for mouth to mouth ventilation and work from the side.
- Tilt the head back with one hand, using the other to support the chin and keep the mouth closed.
- Take a deep breath, seal your mouth around the patient's

nose, and blow through the nose until the chest is seen to rise.

• Passive expiration may be helped by opening the mouth.

Practical point
• Difficulty with inflation may occur with nasal obstruction or a poorly maintained airway.

Babies and infants
• The small face requires the rescuer to seal his mouth around the patient's nose and mouth.

• Smaller breaths will be required to inflate the lungs.

Ventilation: advanced life support (ALS) techniques

The use of simple appliances has a number of advantages. Direct contact between rescuer and patient is avoided and the risk of cross-infection is reduced. Supplemental oxygen may be given and oropharyngeal or nasopharyngeal airways may be used.

Mouth to mask ventilation

This technique is suitable for resuscitation both inside and outside hospital. It is more efficient than poorly performed bag–valve–mask ventilation which should only be used after adequate training.

Technique
• Lay the patient supine, and work from the top (Fig. 8.21).
• Open the airway by the head-tilt method.
• Fit the face mask over the nose and mouth, ensuring a seal all the way round (the tapered end of the mask fits around the nose).
• Apply gentle downward pressure with the thumbs and forefingers of both hands. The little fingers should hook under the angle of the jaw, and the ring and middle

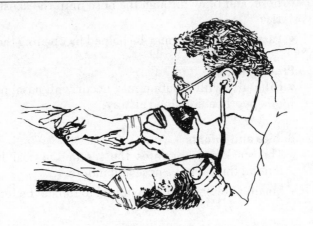

Fig. 8.21 • Mouth to mask ventilation.

fingers should fan forwards under the jaw to secure the hold on the mask. Open the airway by the jaw thrust technique.

- Blow into the mouthpiece of the mask to inflate the chest as if performing mouth to mouth ventilation.

- Supplemental oxygen may be given via the oxygen nipple at a flow-rate of 8 to 10 litres per minute.

Practical points
- Failure to inflate the lungs adequately may be due to a leak around the mask. If this occurs check that the mask is applied correctly and adjust the position of the thumbs and forefingers slightly. An oropharyngeal or a naso-pharyngeal airway may be used if there are problems maintaining the airway.

- This technique could be performed with an ordinary face mask from a self-inflating bag or anaesthetic circuit to avoid direct patient contact. However, supplemental oxygen could not then be given, and there would not be a one-way valve to reduce the risk of infection.

- In small children the mask can be used with the narrow end over the chin and the wider end over the forehead.

- This technique can be practiced on training manikins.

Self-inflating bag/non-rebreathing valve/mask ventilation

This technique uses a manual resuscitator, such as the Laerdal (see p. 42). It has the advantage that high inspired oxygen concentrations can be delivered. Should the patient require intubation, the mask can be removed quickly and the device can be attached to a tracheal tube. The technique cannot be learnt by observation alone. Anyone using the technique must have had adequate training, including practice on training manikins.

Technique

- Lay the patient supine and work from the top (Fig. 8.22).
- Open the airway by head tilt.
- Choose a mask of the correct size and place it over the nose and mouth, with the tapered end over the nose.
- Hold the mask down with the thumb and forefinger of one hand curving around the connector.
- Hook the little finger of the same hand under the angle of the jaw. The ring and middle fingers should fan out under the mandible, and together should lift the jaw in a jaw thrust technique to open the airway.
- Counter-pressure from the thumb and forefinger should ensure an airtight seal.

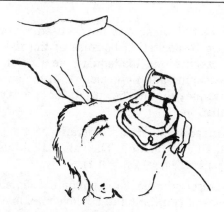

Fig. 8.22 • Bag–valve–mask ventilation.

- Squeeze the bag with the other hand to inflate the lungs.

- After adequate inflation release the bag to allow refilling and passive exhalation through the one-way valve.

- Give oxygen and use an oxygen reservoir bag.

Practical points

- Avoid excessively high flow rates, as this may cause gastric inflation, with subsequent regurgitation and aspiration. This is a particular risk in children.

- If a leak occurs around the mask, check that the mask has been applied correctly and try altering the position of the thumb and forefinger slightly. A good seal may be difficult to maintain, particularly in patients with difficult airways or beards, or in the obese. Rescuers with small hands may also have problems. In this case hold the mask in place with both hands, and get an assistant to squeeze the bag.

- Problems maintaining an airway may be helped by inserting an oropharyngeal or nasopharyngeal airway.

- Rescuers with small hands may find it impossible to expel enough gas from the bag to ventilate a large patient adequately. Ideally two people should then ventilate the patient as described above. If there is no assistant, the rescuer should try squeezing the bag between their palm and either their thigh or a pillow by the patient's head.

- This technique should not be used for prolonged periods during resuscitation because of the risk of regurgitation and aspiration. Inadequate ventilation may result in hypercapnia and hypoxaemia. In the apnoeic patient this technique should be used for preoxygenation before intubation.

- An inspiration–expiration ratio of 1:2 or 1:3 should be used after intubation. The ventilation rate will depend on the patient's age (Table 8.2).

- The reservoir bag must remain inflated throughout all phases of ventilation to achieve maximal inspired oxygen concentrations.

Table 8.2 • Ventilation rates

Patient	Rate (breaths/minute)
Adult	10–12
Child > 2 yrs	12–20
Infant 6 mths–2 yrs	20
Baby < 6 mths	30

Tidal volume = 10–15 ml/kg

Bag–valve–mask ventilation with an anaesthetic breathing system

The breathing system will usually have an expiratory valve, and reservoir bag filling will be dependent on fresh gas flow. Incorrect use or prolonged use with certain systems may cause hypercapnia. This technique should only be used by those with adequate training. The choice of breathing systems is discussed on p. 45. The technique for holding the mask is described above. A two-person technique may be used. Ventilation is likely to be inadequate if:

- there is a leak around the mask
- the expiratory valve is open too far, allowing an excessive leak
- the bag fails to fill because of an inadequate fresh gas flow or a leak from within the breathing system.

During resuscitation this technique should only be used in preparation for intubation. The mask may be removed and the tracheal tube can then be attached to the breathing system. Since there will then be no leaks around the mask, adjustments may be needed to the fresh gas flow rate and valve setting to prevent excessive airways pressure.

Spontaneous ventilation in the intubated patient

If an intubated patient is to breathe spontaneously, the inspired gas mixture must be oxygen-enriched. The patient should be monitored by pulse oximetry and arterial blood gas measurements should be taken. The best system to use is a low resistance T-piece made from corrugated plastic tubing. The length of the expiratory limb of the T-piece determines carbon dioxide retention. If the patient is intubated for a prolonged period the gas mixture must be humidified. If the patient is breathing spontaneously for a brief period an oxygen mask may be held over the end of the tracheal tube but great care must be taken not to occlude the tube or to increase the resistance to breathing.

Mechanical ventilation

Principles of mechanical ventilation

A mechanical ventilator applies an intermittent positive pressure to the airway to overcome the elastic resistance of the lungs and chest wall and the frictional airways resistance. Each ventilatory cycle has four phases: inspiration, cycling from inspiration to expiration, expiration, and cycling from expiration to inspiration.

All ventilators produce an inspiratory flow of gas by developing a pressure gradient between the ventilator and the lungs. A constant pressure generator produces a pressure of 25–30 cm water, causing a flow of gas into the lungs which is affected by lung characteristics. A constant flow generator provides a high enough pressure to give a constant flow of gas into the lungs irrespective of lung characteristics. Mechanical ventilators may also be described in terms of the force applied as 'low pressure' or 'high pressure' ventilators. During inspiration, an increasing volume of gas is delivered to the patient, the pressure in the lungs changes, and the flow alters. Inspiratory wave forms are probably not important. The ventilator cycles from inspiration to expiration when either time, volume, pressure, or flow reaches a preset value. During expiration the ventilator may be pressure or flow generated. Nearly all ventilators operate in expiration as constant pressure generators, allowing a pressure gradient to develop between the final lung pressure and atmospheric pressure. Some ventilators are able to maintain a positive pressure at the end of expiration. The method of cycling from expiration to inspiration may differ from that used to cycle from inspiration to expiration. Time cycling and pressure cycling are the most common. One form of pressure cycling depends upon the patient making an inspiratory effort (patient triggering). Ventilatory modes can be classified as continuous mandatory ventilation (CMV), intermittent mandatory ventilation (IMV), and synchronized intermittent mandatory ventilation (SIMV). Sometimes a mechanical ventilator is used to generate a positive airway pressure in spontaneously breathing patients. Such modes of assistance are called continuous positive airway pressure (CPAP) or pressure support.

Physiological effects of mechanical ventilation

Intermittent positive pressure ventilation (IPPV) alters the distribution of ventilation and perfusion in the lung, increases venous admixture, enlarges physiological dead space, and increases the functional residual capacity. There is a risk of barotrauma, especially in patients with abnormal lungs, which is increased by large tidal volumes, high inflation pressures, and positive end-expiratory pressure (PEEP).

Cardiac output is reduced during IPPV as a result of decreased venous return and external pressure on the left ventricle. The effect of IPPV on cardiac output depends on the patient's cardiorespiratory state. This may be particularly profound in hypovolaemic patients. During IPPV pressure is less well transmitted to the heart and large vessels of patients with stiff lungs. Cardiac function may be improved by ventilation of some patients with severe heart failure.

The increased intrathoracic pressure produced by IPPV reduces renal blood flow, glomerular filtration rate, and urine output, leading to sodium and water retention. The haemodynamic changes produced by IPPV lead to an increased production of antidiuretic hormone, renin, and aldosterone.

Hyperventilation reduces intracranial pressure by reducing arterial carbon dioxide concentrations. This may be useful in the treatment of head injured patients but the effect only lasts for a few hours.

Mechanical ventilation in the A & E setting

Only brief surgical procedures are usually performed under general anaesthesia in the A & E department, and therefore, in most circumstances, patients breathe spontaneously and do not need ventilation. However, ventilators are useful during resuscitation of seriously ill patients both at the scene of accidents and in the hospital. They are also required for the transfer of intubated patients within and outside the hospital.

The choice of a mechanical ventilator

Some of the requirements for a resuscitation ventilator and a machine for use during the transport of critically ill patients are the same. The ventilator should be robust, light, compact, and safe to use. There should be clear instructions printed on the ventilator with controls identifiable in the dark. A time/volume cycled ventilator is preferable. It should have a large inspiratory flow capacity in order to cope with patients with varying lung compliance. It must be suitable for adult or paediatric use. It should have audible pressure relief valves. It should have autoclavable parts and be easy to reassemble after cleaning. It must be reliable in wet or dirty conditions, and should possess an alternative portable power source if there is no gas supply. It should need minimal servicing.

Resuscitation ventilators tend to be used by relatively inexperienced staff. They should be easy to understand and operate and particularly robust, function in adverse circumstances, and supply 100 per cent oxygen. They must not entrain air as this is dangerous if one is rescuing a patient from an adverse environment, for example in the presence of toxic gases.

Ventilators for transferring critically ill patients tend to be used by more experienced staff. Transport ventilators are more sophisticated than ventilators used for resuscitation. They should supply a range of oxygen concentrations by using air entrainment, provide PEEP, monitor airway pressure, and be compatible with heat and moisture exchangers.

Guidelines for mechanical ventilation

The requirements for ventilation depend upon the circumstances. It is not possible to give recommendations for ventilation for all situations, but the following guidelines are suggested:

- If the tidal volume can be set, at least 10 ml/kg should be delivered. Large tidal volumes may be useful in hypo-xaemic patients, but large volumes increase the risk of barotrauma and may reduce cardiac output.

- If the ventilatory frequency can be set, neonates need 30–40 breaths/minute, infants 20 breaths/minute, and adults 10–12 breaths/minute. In certain circumstances changes in ventilatory frequency can improve oxygenation.

- If the minute volume can be set, administer 100–120 ml/kg in adults and 180–200 ml/kg in children.

- Loss of gas due to compression and leaks should be taken into consideration when setting the ventilator.

- If the inspiratory:expiratory (I:E) ratio is variable, adults are usually given a ratio of 1:1 and children 1:2. A longer expiratory time may be needed if there is high airways resistance. Reversed I:E ratios may be useful in hypo-xaemia.

- Inflation pressure should be kept below a peak value of 30 cm water, to minimize the risk of barotrauma. Alterations in ventilatory volumes and timing may be used to reduce the peak and mean inflation pressures.

- PEEP may be employed to improve oxygenation, especially in children but PEEP increases the chance of barotrauma and reduces cardiac output. The potential for adverse effects should be balanced against the possible benefits of improved oxygenation.

- 100 per cent oxygen should be administered during resuscitation; otherwise the oxygen concentration should be set to maintain a normal or slightly high oxygen saturation.

- In the A & E or resuscitation setting the patient is usually fully ventilated, and not allowed to make respiratory efforts to trigger the ventilator.

- If the patient is to be ventilated for a prolonged period a heat and moisture exchanger should be included in the breathing circuit.

Monitoring mechanical ventilation

Circulatory function and gas exchange must be assessed regularly. The following observations are necessary.

- Observation of chest movement, percussion, and ausculta-tion is useful in confirming the adequacy of ventilation. Problems such as bronchial intubation, pneumothorax, and atelectasis may be detectable clinically.

- Regular observation of the patients' colour, peripheral perfusion, heart rate, and blood pressure is essential.

- ECG monitoring is mandatory. Cardiac arrhythmias are a late sign of ventilatory problems. Bradycardia in children suggests hypoxaemia.

- Alveolar ventilation can be monitored using end-tidal or arterial carbon dioxide concentrations. A value of 4.5–5.5 kPa is acceptable, except in a head injured patient, when lower values may be desirable.

- Oxygenation can be assessed by monitoring of trans-cutaneous oxygen saturation; values in excess of 95 per cent are satisfactory. Measurement of arterial oxygen concen-tration is needed, values greater than 10 kPa are acceptable.

- An oxygen analyser should be used to monitor delivered oxygen concentrations.

- If volatile anaesthetic agents are in use the inspired and expired concentrations should be monitored. This is particularly important if low gas flows are in use.

- Monitoring of the mean and peak inflation pressure is use-ful. A sudden increase may reflect a blocked or displaced tracheal tube, bronchospasm, pulmonary oedema, or a pneumothorax.

- A disconnection alarm is mandatory.

Gastric tube insertion

The placement of a gastric tube, via the nose or mouth, should be considered during the resuscitation phase of every major trauma patient. If there are facial injuries or base of skull fracture an oral rather than a nasal tube should be used. A gastric tube should be considered in acute medical and surgical conditions where there is a high risk of regurgitation and aspiration, for example diabetic ketoacidosis or acute intestinal obstruction.

Technique
- Lay the patient supine and choose an appropriately sized, well-lubricated tube.
- Insert the tube into the right nostril and direct it gently through the nostril to the nasopharynx and down the oesophagus into the stomach.
- If the tube will not pass through the right nostril remove it and try the other side.
- Correct placement can be confirmed by using litmus paper to detect gastric acid.
- Secure the tube with adhesive tape, connect it to a collecting bag, and leave it on open drainage.

Practical points
- Never insert a nasogastric tube if the cribiform plate may be fractured, since the tube may be directed up into the intracranial cavity. It may be possible to introduce the tube through the mouth.
- Avoid movement of the head and neck in patients with a suspected cervical spine injury.
- In the conscious patient, passage of the tube into and through the oesophagus may be helped by using lignocaine gel and moving the tube when the patient swallows.
- In the unconscious patient, the tube may be inserted under direct vision, using a laryngoscope and Magill forceps.
- The tube may be easier to pass if it has been stored in a fridge. The cooler plastic is firmer and distorts less during insertion.
- Difficulty directing the tube through the nostril may be overcome using a well-lubricated split nasal tube. This is first introduced into the nostril. The nasogastric tube is passed along it into the nasopharynx and oesophagus. The first tube is then carefully removed without disturbing the nasogastric tube.
- The passage of a gastric tube does not guarantee a safe airway.

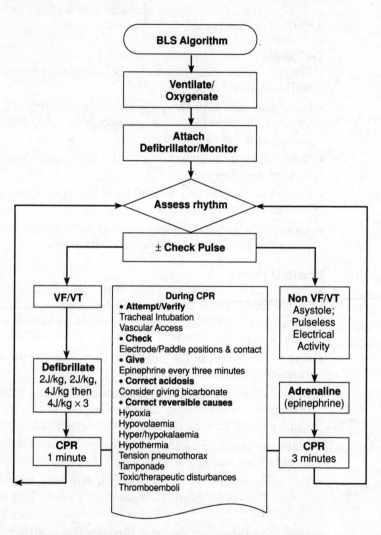

Fig. 8.20 • Paediatric advanced life support guidelines. By kind permission of Resuscitation Council (UK). VF: ventricular fibrillation; VT: ventricular tachycardia; ETT: endotracheal tube; IV: intravenous; CPR: cardiopulmonary resuscitation.

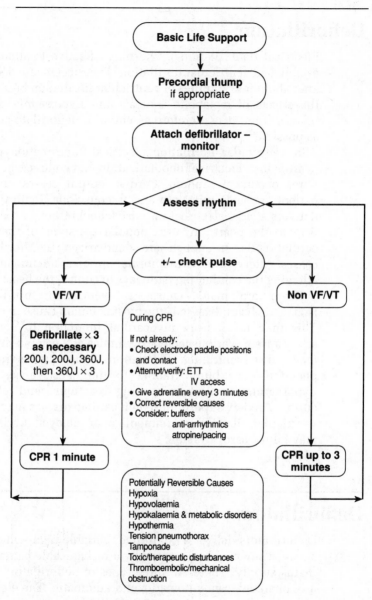

The algorithm is based on the assumption that the previous step was unsuccessful.

Fig. 8.21 • Adult advanced life support guidelines. By kind permission of Resuscitation Council (UK) (1997).

Defibrillation

Electrical defibrillation is the only effective treatment for established ventricular fibrillation. The success rate declines after about four minutes of ventricular fibrillation because of the effects of metabolic acidosis and hypoxaemia on the myocardium. It is therefore essential to defibrillate as soon as possible.

In ventricular fibrillation electrical coordination of the heart is lost. Electrical depolarization and contraction of the fibres occurs at random. Cardiac output ceases and the patient becomes pulseless and unconscious. Defibrillation delivers a large electrical impulse (shock) through the chest wall to the heart, and this depolarizes some of the myocardial cells. If enough are depolarized the fibrillation ceases. After a brief period normal impulses are transmitted, allowing the conducting pathways to control the heart beat.

There are many causes of ventricular fibrillation. Ischaemic heart disease is the most common cause in adults. This may range from myocardial infarction to coronary artery spasm. Various tachyarrhythmias and ectopic rhythms may cause ventricular fibrillation. Other causes include penetrating or blunt trauma to the chest, anaesthesia, hypothermia, hypoxaemia, drug reactions, and electrocution. Anxiety superimposed on cardiac disease may cause ventricular fibrillation. Immediate or delayed fibrillation may follow cardioversion.

Defibrillators

Defibrillators deliver a controlled, variable high-voltage DC shock. They may be powered by a rechargeable battery or a mains supply. There are three types of defibrillator: manually operated, semiautomatic, and automatic. The electrical impulse is delivered through well protected hand-held paddles or electrodes, which have a discharge button. The time to attain maximum charge should be less than 10 seconds with a mains operated or fully charged battery powered unit. This time may be prolonged by a few seconds after repeated battery use. It should be possible to defibrillate three times within one minute. On some machines the ECG may be monitored through the paddles.

Semiautomatic and automatic defibrillators were designed for use by non-medical personnel. The patient's ECG is monitored by large 10 cm electrodes, and interpreted by an integral computer. The machine indicates the presence of ventricular fibrillation and the need to defibrillate. The semi-automatic machine requires an operator to discharge the shock, while the automatic machine does this itself. All machines give audible warnings of imminent defibrillation. When using these machines a period of up to 90 seconds is acceptable to diagnose ventricular fibrillation and deliver three shocks.

Electrical defibrillation is the only effective treament for established ventricular fibrillation. It is essential to defibrillate as soon as possible.

Doctors starting a new job should familiarize themselves with the defibrillators used in the hospital. Doctors caring for children should know the correct settings and paddles to use for paediatric resuscitation.

Some complications of defibrillation can be prevented by attention to technique.

It is essential that meticulous attention to safety is always given during defibrillation.

Indications

Asynchronous shock or defibrillation:

- Ventricular fibrillation
- Pulseless ventricular tachycardia

Synchronized cardioversion:

- Ventricular tachycardia
- Atrial fibrillation
- Paroxysmal atrial tachycardia or junctional tachycardia

Contraindications

- Idiojunctional or idioventricular rhythms
- Second or third degree heart blocks

Precautions

- Do not defibrillate in the presence of flammable agents or anaesthetics.
- Do not discharge the defibrillator
  - (a) with the paddles held together
  - (b) into open air
  - (c) if the paddle handles are wet or covered with gel
  - (d) if any person is touching the patient or any equipment that is in contact with the patient.
- Oxygen because of fire risk (see below).
- Disconnect the patient from equipment which may be damaged by defibrillation, such as external pacing devices.
- Do not defibrillate in the presence of high energy electrical fields, such as those generated by diathermy. The diathermy must be turned off first.
- Remove glyceryl trinitrate and other skin patches before defibrillation.

Technique

Defibrillation forms part of the advanced life support protocol (see p. 178, 179).

- Apply gel pads. The standard position is with the right pad to the right of the sternum just below the clavicle and the left pad over the fifth left intercostal space in the midclavicular line.
- Select the correct paddles (during charging the paddles should either be secure in the defibrillator or held on the gel pads applied to the patient's chest).
- Select the required energy and clearly tell personnel 'defibrillator charging'.
- Press the charge button (on the paddle or the defibrillator control panel).
- Wait until the defibrillator is charged.
- Ensure that the paddle electrodes are placed correctly on the gel pads.
- Shout 'stand back'.

- Check that all personnel and yourself are clear.
- Deliver the shock by passing the discharge buttons on the paddles simultaneously.
- Check the pulse for five seconds to see if cardiac output has been restored.

Fires from defibrillation during oxygen administration

Patients and their bedding have been set on fire during defibrillation. This has occurred when oxygen, used in resuscitation, produced an oxygen enriched space around the patient's head and chest which allowed an electric arc, produced during defibrillation, to ignite body hair. An electric arc can be produced if there is poor interface between the defibrillator paddles and the patient's skin.

Defibrillation performed in the presence of oxygen does not typically result in fire but if the localized oxygen concentration is significantly above ambient in the vicinity of the paddles a flash fire may result. Fires during defibrillation can be prevented by:

- Minimizing the presence of oxygen-enriched spaces around the patient's head and upper body. All sources of supplemental oxygen must be removed from the area around the patient before defibrillation. This includes all manual and gas-powered resuscitators, breathing circuits, masks, and nasal cannulae that provide more than 21 per cent oxygen. Do not leave such devices near the patient or on the bed during defibrillation.

- Reducing the chance of arcing by establishing a good contact between the paddles and the patient's skin. The defibrillator paddles should be applied while ensuring even and unobstructed contact with the disposable gel pads. ECG electrodes should be as far away from the paddles as possible. Defibrillator paddles should not be placed on the ECG electrode or wire (Hazard Report 1994).

Practical points
- It is essential to maintain oxygenation using routine cardiac life support. Hypoxaemia and metabolic acidosis reduce the success of defibrillation. Cardiac compression performed during the establishment of a coordinated

rhythm, following defibrillation, is unlikely to precipitate a recurrence of fibrillation.

- The operator must know how to use the defibrillator before using it for the first time.

- The defibrillator is potentially dangerous to personnel around the patient. Ensure that all persons, including the operator, are not in electrical contact with the patient during defibrillation.

- Synchronized mode should not be used for ventricular fibrillation, since there are no 'R' waves, and these are required for the synchronized mode. Defibrillation would thus be delayed indefinitely.

- Current flow is determined by the shock 'strength' and the thoracic impedance. The latter may be increased by inadequate electrode–chest wall interface, inadequate electrode position, excessive disturbance between electrodes, inadequate electrode pressure, or a pneumothorax.

- Defibrillator contact pads are preferable to electrode jelly, since the latter tends to spread around the chest, which may cause arcing between the electrodes, surface burning of the patient's chest, and failure to defibrillate. This may also occur if the patient's chest is wet, as in cases of near-drowning.

- Ensure that the defibrillator pads never overlap, since this will produce arcing.

- Always use a conductive medium between electrodes and the skin to prevent skin burns. Ensure that all the surface of the electrode is in contact with the gel or jelly. Saline pads may be used if conductive gel pads or jelly are not available.

- Gel pads dry out with use and lose their conductivity. They should be changed after 10 discharges.

- Keep defibrillator paddles clean. Wet or dry gel on the electrode handles produces the risk of electrocution of the operator.

- Adult- and child-size paddles are available. The child paddle often fastens on to the adult paddle.

- Glyceryl trinitrate skin patches should be removed before defibrillating to avoid the risk of arcing between the electrode and the patch.

- A brief period of asystole may occur after defibrillation. Continue ventilation and cardiac compression during this time.

Failed defibrillation

It is essential to maintain oxygenation and prevent acidosis by efficient ventilation and cardiac compression. It might be useful to try using another defibrillator or place the paddles anteriorly and posteriorly. The anterior paddle is placed at the fifth intercostal space in the mid-clavicular line and the posterior paddle is placed just below the inferior angle of the left scapula. Causes of failed defibrillation are listed below.

1. Due to the patient having:
- hypoxaemia
- metabolic acidosis
- myocardial ischaemia
- electrolyte imbalance
- drugs, such as digoxin or bupivacaine toxicity
- hypothermia
- pneumothorax.

2. Due to technique:
- inadequate basic life support
- inadequate energy level
- incorrect paddle position
- inadequate paddle pressure
- shorting of paddles
- forgetting to recharge the defibrillator
- attempting to discharge the paddles before the selected energy level is obtained
- failure to press the discharge buttons simultaneously.

3. Due to the defibrillator:
- the battery level is low and needs recharging
- the 'synchronize' button has been pressed, and in the absence of 'R' waves the defibrillator cannot discharge

- the charge has been dumped as a result of changes made to the 'energy select' dial after the charge was initiated
- in synchronized mode the patient is not being monitored through the patient cable.

Complications of cardioversion

Complications potentially associated with poor technique include:

- skin burns
- arcing
- electrocution
- failed cardioversion
- post-shock arrhythmias.

Those associated with underlying disease include:

- post-shock arrhythmias
- congestive heart failure
- transient hypotension
- pulmonary embolism.

Myocardial injury

Although this has been demonstrated in dogs using repeated high energy shocks, cardioversion performed in the usual manner does not appear to cause any significant damage in humans.

Children

Choose the appropriate size of electrode paddle. In some designs these clip on to the adult paddle. A charge of 2 J/kg should be used for the first two shocks. If unsuccessful the charge may be increased to 4 J/kg. The defibrillator may have special controls to obtain low energy levels. Defibrillator conductive pads may be cut to size to cover the smaller electrode surface. Ensure that the pads never overlap.

Pregnancy

A pregnant patient may require defibrillation like any other patient, since without correction both mother and fetus may die. The standard protocol for defibrillation may be used. Aortocaval compression must be avoided.

Pacemakers

Alteration in pacemaker programming or a change in cardiac stimulation threshold may occur following defibrillation. Pacemaker failure has also been described. The following recommendations for defibrillation of a patient with a pacemaker have been made:

• Use low energy, infrequent DC shock.

• Place the paddles in a line perpendicular to the pacer axis (ideally anterior–posterior).

• Place the paddles at least 10 cm from the electrodes and the pulse generator.

• Check the pacemaker function after defibrillation (some units will reset to a predetermined set of values).

• Have emergency pacing equipment available.

Further reading

American College of Surgeons (1993). *Advanced trauma life support program for physicians*. American College of Surgeons, Chicago.

European Resuscitation Council (1992). *Resuscitation*, **22**, 111–21.

European Resuscitation Council (1996). *Resuscitation*, **31**, 187–230. Published by Elsevir Science Ireland, Ltd., Shannon Industrial Estate, C. Clare, Ireland.

Gray, A. G. J. (1981). Portable lung ventilators. *British Journal of Hospital Medicine*, **25**, 173–8.

Harries, M. G. (1983). Portable lung ventilators under field conditions. *Anaesthesia*, **38**, 279–81.

Hazard Report (1994). Fires from defibrillation during oxygen administration. *Health Devices*, **23**, 307–8.

Oakley, P. A., Phillips, B., Molyneux, E. and Mackway-Jones, K. (1993). Updated standard reference chart. *British Medical Journal*, **306**, 1613.

Park, G. R., Manara, A. R., Bodenham, A. R., and Moss, C. J. (1989). The pneuPAC ventilator with new patient valve and air compressors. *Anaesthesia*, **44**, 419–24.

Phillips, G. D. and Stowonski, G.A. (1986). Manual respirators and portable ventilators. *Anaesthesia and Intensive Care*, **14**, 306–13.

Resuscitation Council (UK) (1997). *The 1997 resuscitation guidelines for use in the United Kingdom*.

Weg, J. G. and Haas, C. F. (1989). Safe intrahospital transfer of critically ill , ventilator dependent patients. *Chest*, **96**, 631–5.

Williams, K. N. and Nunn, J. F. (1989). The oesophageal detector device. *Anaesthesia*, **44**, 412–14.

Zideman, D. A. (1995). Resuscitation of infants and children. In *ABC of Resuscitation*, Ed. Colquhoun, M. C. Handley, A. J. and Evans, T. R. BMJ Publishing Group.

Advanced trauma life support courses

These are advertised in the medical journals or information may be obtained from

The Royal College of Surgeons of England,
35–43 Lincoln's Inn Fields,
London WC2A 3PN.

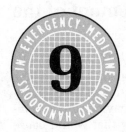

CHAPTER 9

Common problems in airway and ventilation management

Key points in common problems in airway and ventilation management

- Any patient with depressed consciousness is at risk of airway obstruction, ventilatory depression, and aspiration of gastric contents.
- Airway or breathing problems may cause hypoxaemia. Adequate oxygenation is essential.
- Asthma may be fatal if the severity is underestimated or treatment is inadequate.
- Respiratory arrest in children may be due to infection, poisoning, trauma, or inhalation of a foreign body.
- Most chest injuries can be treated with oxygen, chest drainage, fluid replacement, and analgesia.
- Head injured patients deteriorate if hypoxaemic or hypercapnic. It is essential to maintain a patent airway and adequate ventilation with oxygen.
- Spinal cord injury may cause hypoventilation.
- Airway obstruction may develop rapidly in a patient with stridor after a thermal injury. Inhalation of steam is especially likely to cause airway problems. Thermal injury is particularly dangerous in children.

Initial assessment and management of the airway

Inadequate airway control may rapidly lead to asphyxia and death. Unconsciousness and obstruction or injury to the upper respiratory tract are the main factors causing hypoxaemia and death. A conscious patient may be able to compensate for a partially obstructed airway that would cause hypoxaemia in a patient with an impaired consciousness level. It is easy to diagnose an airway problem when the patient is cyanosed and has blood bubbling from a distorted face. A more difficult problem is presented by the patient with impaired conciousness who quietly regurgitates and aspirates gastric contents, and then develops hypoxaemic brain damage.

Any patient with a depressed consciousness from any cause is at risk of developing airway obstruction, aspiration of gastric contents, or ventilatory depression. The risk is increased if the patient has recently received an opioid. The intramuscular route may be particularly hazardous because of unpredictable absorption, especially in the shocked patient. Analgesics should be used where indicated but they should be given in carefully controlled intravenous doses, with adequate resuscitation equipment available. Naloxone should also be available to reverse the ventilatory depressant effect of opioids. For further discussion see p. 242.

Guidelines for the assessment of the airway and ventilation are given in Fig. 9.1. Patients with airway problems require added oxygen. Give 100 per cent oxygen and monitor by oximetry, supplemented by arterial blood gas estimation. Capnography may also be useful to monitor the efficiency of ventilation. Tables 9.1–9.3 list the range of causes of airway obstruction, stridor in children, and hypoventilation.

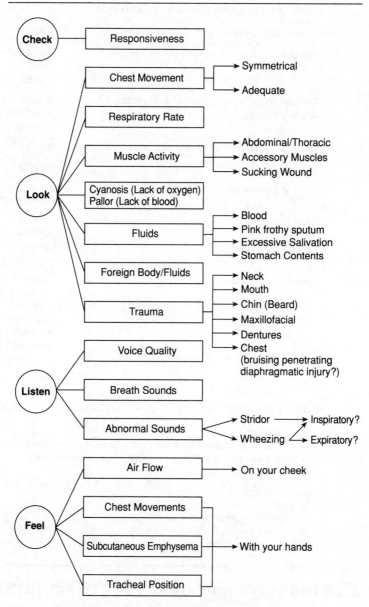

Fig. 9.1 ● Assessment of the airway and ventilation, according to European Resuscitation Council (ERC) guideline (1996). By kind permission of ERC and Elsevier Science Ireland Ltd.

Table 9.1 • Causes of airway obstruction

Type of obstruction	Cause
Occlusion of the oropharynx by the tongue	cardiac arrest coma trauma
Tongue oedema, oropharynx obstruction, laryngeal spasm	anaphylaxis foreign body irritants/burns
Laryngeal, tracheal, or bronchial obstruction	foreign body
Laryngeal damage	trauma
Laryngeal oedema	anaphylaxis infection/burns
Bronchospasm	anaphylaxis asthma foreign body irritants/burns
Pulmonary oedema	anaphylaxis cardiac failure infection irritants/burns near-drowning neurogenic shock

Table 9.2 • Common causes of respiratory distress in children

Upper airway:
- loss of consciousness – head injury, during or after convulsion
- infection – croup, epiglottitis, laryngotracheo-bronchitis
- inhaled foreign body

Lower airway:
- asthma
- infective – bronchiolitis, pneumonia
- inhaled foreign body

The management of stridor in children

Stridor in a child is an emergency. Senior anaesthetic and paediatric assistance should be summoned urgently. Children deteriorate quickly if the airway is obstructed, for the following reasons.

Table 9.3 • Causes of hypoventilation

Central depression due to
- hypoxaemia
- hypercapnia
- hypotension
- poisoning
- head injury
- electrocution

Failure of efferent nerve supply in
- spinal cord injury
- polyneuritis
- neuropathy

Respiratory muscle failure due to
- electrolyte or acid–base disturbance
- muscle-relaxant drugs
- obesity
- myasthenia gravis
- muscular dystrophy

Thoracic injury
- tension pneumothorax
- haemothorax
- flail chest
- ruptured diaphragm
- severe burns of chest wall

Voluntary restriction of ventilatory effort
- pain – fractured ribs, peritonitis, post-operative

- Air flow through the trachea is proportional to the fourth power of its radius. A small reduction in the diameter of the trachea, for example as a result of oedema, produces a large change in air flow. Alterations in tracheal diameter in children have a proportionately greater effect than in adults because of the small size of the trachea.

- In children the mucosa of the larynx is only loosely attached anteriorly and along the aryepiglottic folds. Any supraglottic oedema forces the epiglottis to curl backwards over the laryngeal inlet and obstruct the airway.

- Young children have a relatively soft trachea, which is more easily compressed than that of an adult.

Assessment

The history and clinical examination of the child form the most important aspect of assessment of airway obstruction.

The history may suggest a congenital problem, an infection, or inhalation of a foreign body. Tachypnoea is often the first sign of ventilatory distress in infants. Increased ventilatory rate and pulse rate are useful signs of deterioration (a ventilatory rate of more than 60 breaths per minute in an infant and 40 breaths per minute in an older child should cause concern). Restlessness is an important sign of worsening airway obstruction. Oximetry is a useful non-invasive monitor. Blood gas changes are a late manifestation of airway obstruction. Bradycardia in a distressed child is a very ominous sign.

Causes of stridor

- Congenital (cystic hygroma, laryngomalacia, vascular rings, laryngeal cysts, and laryngeal webs)
- Trauma (tracheal injury, burns, ingestion of caustic substances, and a story of traumatic or prolonged intubation leading to subglottic oedema or stenosis)
- Infection (acute epiglottitis, large tonsils, a retropharyngeal abscess, laryngotracheo-bronchitis (croup), and diphtheria)
- A foreign body
- Angioneurotic oedema
- Laryngeal tumours (papillomata or subglottic haemangiomata)

Immediate management

- The child must be observed constantly for signs of worsening airway obstruction. A child should not be upset, as crying increases the difficulty in breathing. Separation from the parent, physical examination, or venepuncture must be avoided until the necessary personnel and equipment are available for intubation.
- The child is often best kept sitting and, if possible, breathing oxygen held by a parent. Monitoring the oxygen saturation is useful, if the child is not upset by this.
- A senior paediatrician, senior anaesthetist, and senior throat surgeon should be called.

- Sedatives should NEVER be given to a child with stridor.

- Nebulized racemic adrenaline may be helpful in post-extubation stridor or croup. The usual dose is 0.25–0.5 ml of 2.25 per cent racemic adrenaline for all age groups, this is equivalent to approximately 5 mg of L-adrenaline. There is no place for the use of nebulized adrenaline in the treatment of acute epiglottitis.

- If the airway obstruction is severe, intubation can provide prolonged airway control. Tracheostomy is only rarely indicated, although it is helpful to have a surgeon present. Intubation of a child with stridor should only be attempted by an experienced anaesthetist. Skilled assistance, a selection of laryngoscopes, tracheal tubes, and other aids to intubation should be available. Gaseous induction of anaesthesia using a volatile agent in 100 per cent oxygen is the safest method. Airway obstruction may increase as anaesthesia deepens. The use of continuous positive airways pressure early during induction of anaesthesia is helpful. Muscle relaxants are contraindicated unless the anaesthetist is sure that oxygenation can be maintained. An oral tracheal tube may be passed in the first instance, it may be replaced by a nasal tracheal tube. The tracheal tube should be secured carefully. Spontaneous breathing of humidified oxygen-enriched air is usually most appropriate. Some children need ventilation.

- Once the airway is secure, venous access must be established. Prolonged airway obstruction may cause dehydration. Excessive fluid administration must be avoided as this may lead to pulmonary oedema.

- Steroids such as budesonide are useful in croup. Intravenous dexamethasone (0.25 mg/kg initially and then 0.1 mg/kg every 6 h for 24 h) may be helpful in post-extubation stridor. Steroids have no place in the immediate management of epiglottitis.

- If the cause of the stridor is infection, an appropriate antibiotic should be administered.

- The child must be transferred to an intensive care unit.

Ventilatory failure in the A & E department

There are many causes of ventilatory failure. Those more commonly seen in the A & E department include

- chest disease: chronic obstructive airway disease, asthma;
- major trauma: head, thoracic, or spinal injury;
- cardiac arrest;
- inhalation: vomit, smoke, chemicals;
- drug overdose.

The anaesthetist will be involved with patients requiring tracheal intubation and ventilation. Some patients will already be intubated and ventilated as part of their primary resuscitation. Patients with severe chronic obstructive airways disease or asthma may need ventilation, which may also be required to prevent deterioration of the patient's condition following severe head injury or airway burns.

The decision to ventilate a patient may be difficult but delay can be fatal. Early consultation with an anaesthetist is advisable. The junior anaesthetist may need time to consult with senior colleagues and to arrange transfer to the intensive care unit when the patient's condition has stabilized. Many patients with chronic obstructive airways disease or asthma will be known to the hospital. If necessary the case should be discussed with the patient's general practitioner and consultant physician. Paediatricians must always be involved in the management of children with ventilatory failure. Relevant medical information must be obtained quickly, since this may avoid inappropriate management.

Acute exacerbation of chronic obstructive airways disease

Infection is the most common cause of an acute exacerbation of chronic chest disease but the chest must be examined carefully to exclude other causes. Primary treatment consists of controlled oxygen therapy, initially 24 per cent oxygen, with nebulized salbutamol 5 mg and ipratropium 0.5 mg. Response is monitored by observation, serial blood gas estimations, and peak expiratory flow (PEF) measurements. Further management may include the use of steroids, an aminophylline infusion, appropriate antibiotics, and a doxapram infusion. Doxapram may be required if the Pa_{O_2} remains <6 kPa or the Pa_{CO_2} rises by >1.5 kPa despite treatment. Failure to improve the patient's condition may be due to a pneumothorax, pneumonia, pulmonary embolism, sputum plugging, pulmonary oedema, or sedative drugs. These conditions must be treated as appropriate. Mechanical ventilation may be required if there is no response to doxapram. The decision to institute mechanical ventilation must be reached after carefully considering the patient's past medical history, assessing the patient's chest clinically, looking at how tired the patient has become, and considering the trends in the blood gases. Ventilation is relatively contraindicated if previous exercise capacity was severely limited. The circumstances regarding any previous elective ventilation must also be considered.

Acute asthma

Avoidable deaths from asthma still occur. Guidelines exist for the management of asthma (British Thoracic Society and others 1993). The severity of an attack should not be underestimated. A patient with acute severe or life-threatening asthma may not be distressed and may not have the abnormalities commonly associated with the problem.

A patient with acute severe asthma may be too breathless to talk, with a respiratory rate of ≥25 breaths/min (≥50 breaths/min in a child) and a pulse rate of ≥110 beats/min (≥140 beats/min in a child). The peak expiratory flow (PEF) is often ≤50 per cent of the predicted value. Nebulized salbutamol 5 mg or terbutaline 10 mg with 40–60 per cent oxygen as the driving gas should be given immediately. Prednisolone tablets 30–60 mg (1–2 mg/kg body weight to a maximum of 40 mg for children) or intravenous hydrocortisone 200 mg (100 mg for children) should be given, and the patient should be admitted to hospital. Careful monitoring is required since further treatment may be needed. Arterial blood gas estimation is necesary to assess the severity of the attack. Pulse oximetry is also useful to monitor the response to treatment.

Features of life-threatening asthma include exhaustion, confusion, agitation, reduced consciousness, or coma. There may be cyanosis, a silent chest, or poor respiratory effort. Bradycardia or hypotension may occur. The PEF, if recordable, is $\leqslant 33$ per cent of the predicted or best value. Arterial blood gas estimation will show a normal (5–6 kPa) or high Pa_{CO_2}, severe hypoxia ($Pa_{O_2} < 8$ kPa) irrespective of oxygen treatment, and a low pH. A patient with life-threatening asthma requires immediate oxygen, salbutamol, or terbutaline and hydrocortisone as described for acute severe asthma. In addition, ipratropium 0.5 mg, (0.25 mg for a child or 0.125 mg for an infant) should be added to the salbutamol or terbutaline. Intravenous aminophylline may be required and caution is needed when giving a bolus of aminophylline if the patient is already taking theophyllines. Intravenous salbutamol or terbutaline may be used in adults. Chest radiography is necessary to exclude a pneumothorax.

Admission to the intensive care unit will generally be required for a patient with life- threatening asthma or when there is deterioration of acute severe asthma, such as worsening or persistent hypoxaemia, or hypercarbia and a deteriorating PEF. Occasionally patients require mechanical ventilation.

Tracheal intubation and mechanical ventilation of patients with high airways resistance is fraught with danger. There is a high incidence of barotrauma, with pneumothorax and pneumomediastinum. Patients must be deeply sedated before intubation to prevent reflex bronchospasm in response to manipulation of the airway. Slow rates of ventilation with a long expiratory phase may be helpful in reducing peak and mean airway pressures. If sudden deterioration occurs during mechanical ventilation of asthmatic patients, pneumothoraces must be assumed, and the chest must be drained on both sides if necessary. This should not be delayed by waiting for a chest radiograph to confirm the diagnosis.

Severe head injury

A patient with a severe head injury is at risk of tentorial herniation (coning). This is caused by a rise in intracranial pressure which may be due to an enlarging intracranial haematoma or cerebral oedema. Hypoxaemia, hypercapnia, convulsions, hyperthermia, and hyperglycaemia exacerbate the situation. Ratings such as the Glasgow coma scale (GCS) were developed to help reduce ambiguity in the description of patients with alterations in consciousness level. Numerical rating also allows development of management protocols. A patient with no eye opening (E1), inability to follow commands (M1–5), and no word verbalization (V1–2) has a GCS of 8 or less, and a severe head injury.

These patients require 100 per cent oxygen through a clear airway. Fluids containing glucose must be avoided. The GCS, ventilatory rate, pulse rate, and blood pressure should be recorded regularly. Blood gas measurements are required. The anaesthetist should be called early in cases where intubation and ventilation of the patient may be required, or if convulsions occur. Convulsions may be treated with intravenous Diazemuls or thiopentone. Diazemuls may cause ventilatory depression requiring mechanical ventilation. Thiopentone should only be used if tracheal intubation is planned. Hypoxaemia and hypercapnia may be due to chest injuries. If primary treatment of chest problems does not produce an improvement then mechanical ventilation may be required.

Signs of worsening condition and imminent coning include a deterioration in GCS, increased blood pressure, and decreased pulse rate and ventilatory rate. Immediate tracheal intubation, mechanical ventilation, and intravenous mannitol, 0.5 g/kg, are needed. Diuretics are sometimes used. A urinary catheter should be passed. A neurosurgical opinion must be obtained urgently, since the patient may require a CT scan, transfer to a neurosurgical unit, or immediate surgery.

Hypercapnia affects the cerebral circulation by causing cerebral vaso-dilatation which increases the intracranial blood volume and pressure. Hyperventilation induces hypocapnia, which has the converse effects. Maintenance of a Pa_{CO_2} of 3.5 kPa is thought to be beneficial to severely head injured patients, but the effect may only persist for a few hours.

The stimulation from tracheal intubation may produce a significant rise in intracranial pressure. Intubation must be performed smoothly, with appropriate anaesthesia and muscle relaxation. At no time must a patient be allowed to struggle against laryngoscopy or cough on the tracheal tube. The possibility of a neck injury must always be remembered during intubation.

Spinal cord injury

Hypoventilation may occur with paralysis of the intercostal muscles after an injury to the upper thoracic or lower cervical spinal cord. The diaphragm will also be paralysed after injury to the middle or upper cervical cord, and this will cause severe ventilatory failure. A conscious patient will be able to identify pain at the site of injury. A high degree of suspicion is needed in the unconscious patient. An unconscious patient with injuries resulting from a fall or a road traffic accident has a 5–10 per cent chance of having a spinal cord injury. Signs which may be helpful in diagnosing such a lesion include

- hypotension with bradycardia, especially without hypovolaemia
- grimaces to painful stimuli above but not below the clavicle
- ability to flex but not to extend at the elbow
- diaphragmatic breathing
- flaccid areflexia, especially with a flaccid rectal sphincter
- priapism.

Tracheal intubation and ventilation will be required if there are signs of ventilatory failure and particularly when there are associated head or chest injuries. Intubation must be performed with the neck fully immobilized to prevent exacerbation of any spinal cord injury (see p. 155).

Total spinal immobilization is required for patients with a suspected or proven spinal injury. The cervical spine should be immobilized by manual in-line immobilization until a spinal board with head immobilizer can be applied. The spine should be immobilized until a fracture has been excluded.

Thoracic injury

Relatively few patients with chest injuries need a thoractomy. Most can be treated with oxygen, fluid replacement, and chest drainage. Response can be monitored with serial records of vital signs, pulse oximetry, and arterial blood gas measurements. The anaesthetist should be involved early. Assistance with airway management may be given, or the patient may require anaesthesia for operative treatment of associated injuries. Multiple rib fractures may be managed on the intensive care unit using thoracic epidural or intrapleural analgesia. Occasionally, tracheal intubation and ventilation may be necessary, if the patient remains hypoxaemic or develops distress. Patients with pulmonary contusion, with or without a flail chest, are more likely to require mechanical ventilation. Other factors which predispose to the need for early ventilation include impaired consciousness level, abdominal injury producing ileus or requiring laparotomy, skeletal injury requiring immobilization, and pre-existing pulmonary disease.

Cardiac arrest in adults

Ventricular fibrillation is the most common cause of cardiac arrest in adults. The definitive treatment is defibrillation but patients are often intubated and ventilated as part of the resuscitation procedure. In some patients spontaneous respiration does not return immediately, despite restoration of adequate cardiac output. This may be due to cerebral hypoxaemia or oedema. Ventilation may be depressed by previously administered opioids, particularly if they are given intramuscularly. Mechanical ventilation must continue if the patient is unconscious, has severe pulmonary problems, or is hypoxaemic—Pa_{O_2} <9 kPa (on 60 per cent oxygen) or Pa_{CO_2} >6.5 kPa. Hypoxaemia may be due to oesophageal or bronchial intubation, pulmonary oedema, inhalation of vomit, pulmonary embolism, pneumonia, or pneumothorax. The patient must have regained active laryngeal reflexes and be breathing adequately before extubation is attempted. Shallow, infrequent ventilation occurs in some patients after cardiac arrest and premature extubation at this stage may be followed by a ventilatory arrest requiring re-intubation. Oxygen must be administered after the patient is extubated, and oxygenation should be monitored.

Ventilatory arrest in children

Ventilatory arrest in children may be due to infection, such as meningitis, septicaemia, chest infection, or gastro-enteritis; to poisoning; to inhalation of a foreign body; or to major trauma. The anaesthetist's role in poisoning is discussed on p. 204. Management of inhaled foreign bodies is described on p. 136. Emergency management of a child with a ventilatory or cardiac arrest follows the standard protocol for basic and advanced life support. Inexperience in managing a child necessitates early assistance from the paediatrician and the anaesthetist, who can help with airway management, venous access, drug dosage, and initial investigations and diagnosis. Mechanical ventilation must continue if the patient remains unconscious or hypoxaemic. Occasionally a small child may require elective ventilation to manage ventilatory failure secondary to a chest infection. This decision must be shared between the paediatrician and anaesthetist.

Inhalation

Smoke

Patients who have been in an enclosed space during a fire are at risk of upper airway and pulmonary complications. Clinical features include altered consciousness level, direct burns to the face or oropharynx, drooling of saliva, dysphagia, soot in nostrils or sputum, hoarseness, stridor, and expiratory wheeze.

Stridor, difficulty in swallowing, a hoarse voice, and drooling of saliva are signs of epiglottic swelling. An anaesthetist should be called immediately because early tracheal intubation may be required. If intubation is unsuccessful or complete airway obstruction occurs a cricothyroidotomy is required.

All patients with suspected smoke or thermal injury to the respiratory tract should be given humidified high flow oxygen (at least 40–60 per cent) by face mask. Bronchospasm should be treated with a nebulized agonist such as salbutamol or terbutaline.

The airway and ventilation should be reassessed frequently. Increasing respiratory rate could indicate the onset of ventilatory failure. Serial measurements of arterial blood gas tensions, carboxyhaemoglobin, and peak expiratory flow rate (if the patient can comply) should be taken. Pulse oximetry may give erroneous readings due to the presence of carboxyhaemoglobin. Carbon particles in the sputum and a high blood carboxyhaemoglobin concentration should alert staff that lung damage may be present. Ventilatory failure following smoke inhalation is indicated by an increasing respiratory rate and dyspnoea.

Ventilatory support may be indicated when

- respiration rate >30/min
- vital capacity <12–15 ml/kg
- Pa_{O_2} <11.0 kPa (on 40 per cent oxygen)
- Pa_{O_2} <6.0 kPa (on air)
- Pa_{CO_2} high enough to cause a fall in pH to 7.2 (Langford and Armstrong 1989)

The patient requires nasotracheal intubation and admission to the intensive care unit. When severe hypoxaemia occurs with adequate spontaneous ventilation (Pa_{CO_2} <6 kPa) continuous positive airway pressure by mask may be effective. Venous access for both intravenous therapy and central venous pressure monitoring, if necessary, should be established early. Treatment with hyperbaric oxygen may be indicated in patients with carboxyhaemoglobinaemia, particularly if they are or have been unconscious, have cardiac or neurological symptoms, or are pregnant. Early consultation with the local hyperbaric oxygen specialist is advisable.

Other toxic gases produced at the fire may cause problems. Always check that deterioration is not due to thick circumferential chest burns restricting ventilation. These will need urgent escharotomy.

Steam

Inhalation of steam is much more likely to cause airway problems than inhalation of smoke. Thermal injury is especially dangerous in children. Cases have been reported of children who have inhaled steam from a teapot spout and developed laryngeal obstruction. If steam inhalation is suspected from the history or from evidence of scalds around the mouth, the buccal mucosa, or the tongue, the trachea should be intubated early. Laryngeal oedema develops quickly and is potentially lethal in this situation.

Vomit
Aspiration of gastric contents may provoke bronchspasm and hypoxaemia and also cause a pneumonitis or pneumonia. The treatment is discussed on p. 113.

The poisoned patient

Anaesthetic help may be needed in the management of poisoned patients. Ventilatory depression may occur following opioid, tricyclic antidepressant, or other drug. There may be a reduced ventilatory rate, hypoxaemia, depressed consciousness ingestion, and reduced peripheral perfusion. The basic principles of airway and breathing management should be observed and oxygen should be given. Anaesthetic help should be obtained. Opioid induced hypoventilation can be reversed with naloxone; but the duration of action of most opioids is greater than that of naloxone, which must therefore be given by repeated doses or a continuous infusion. Careful observation of consciousness and breathing must be maintained. Arterial blood gas measurements should be taken. Transfer to an intensive care unit is required if a rapid, sustained improvement in breathing is not achieved, since mechanical ventilation may be required. Children with alcohol intoxication should be carefully monitored, since coma and hypoglycaemia may occur.

Gastric lavage, should only be considered if the patient has taken a life-threatening amount of poison within the previous hour or is deeply unconscious because of poisoning. Lavage should not be used for poisoning with corrosives or petrol except rarely in severe poisoning on specialist advice. Gastric lavage may cause hypoxaemia, aspiration pneumonia, and occasionally oesophageal perforation. Lavage must only be done if there is an adequate cough reflex or the airway is protected by a cuffed tracheal tube. The anaesthetist should advise regarding the need for tracheal intubation to protect the airway. Resuscitation equipment and adequate help must be immediately available when tracheal intubation is attempted. The patient should be preoxygenated and oxygenation should be monitored with an oximeter. Drugs are rarely needed to aid tracheal intubation. It may be necessary to leave the tracheal tube in place until the patient regains protective reflexes.

The unconscious patient

The common causes of coma seen in the A & E department are

- cardiorespiratory arrest
- poisoning: alcohol or drugs
- stroke
- head injury
- hypoglycaemia
- epilepsy

The anaesthetist may be involved with those patients requiring intubation and ventilation. All unconscious patients require the same basic airway management and 100 per cent oxygen should be given. Manual ventilation with a bag and mask or tracheal intubation may be required. Immediate tracheal intubation is needed if the gag reflex is absent. Some patients with ventilatory problems or head injury may require tracheal intubation. All patients needing emergency intubation must be assumed to have a full stomach and to be at risk of regurgitation.

Patient transfer

Ten thousand patients with a life-threatening illness are transported between hospitals annually in the United Kingdom. An anaesthetist is in attendance in about 92 per cent of the cases. A concentration of resources within regional units will increase the number of transfers. Life-threatening complications may occur during transfer, the commonest being hypoxaemia and hypotension. Adequate personnel, resuscitation equipment, and monitoring are essential. There should be supplementary oxygen, suction, emergency drugs, and intravenous fluids available and the capacity to ventilate patients. A cardiac monitor and pulse oximeter are necessary. Cross-matched blood should also accompany the patient as required.

The need to transfer a patient to another unit depends on the patient's injuries and the ability of the first hospital to treat them. The doctor initiates the transfer, which must be agreed by both referring and receiving doctors. Good communication is essential to facilitate efficient transfer. The receiving doctor should be readily available for consultation at all times, and is helped if the referring doctor gives a clear history of the problems and statement of the need for transfer. This should include the patient's name and age, a brief history of the accident, and a summary of the initial findings and response to treatment. When transfer has been agreed, transporting personnel must be notified, indicating any special equipment which may be required. Copies of the patient's initial notes, observation and treatment charts, and radiographs and laboratory results must accompany the patient. Provision must also be made for the transfer of any accompanying relatives. They should not usually travel in the ambulance with the patient.

Emergency treatment during transfer is limited and difficult. It is therefore essential to ensure that the patient's condition is as stable as possible before transfer.

Airway

- Insert an airway or tracheal tube if necessary. If the latter is used it must be very carefully secured to prevent displacement during transfer. Drugs and equipment for reintubation must be available during the journey.

- Administer 100 per cent oxygen.

- Have suction available.

- Insert a nasogastric tube if possible to reduce the risk of aspiration. Ensure that it is well secured and leave it on free drainage.

Breathing

- Provide mechanical ventilation if required, either manually or with a portable ventilator (see p. 175).

Fig. 9.2 • Heimlich valve.

- Insert a chest drain if necessary, and secure it carefully. It is inappropriate to use underwater drainage for transfer. The bottles should be replaced by Heimlich valves, ensuring that they are connected the correct way round (Fig. 9.2). A chest drainage bag with a built in flap valve may also be used. Spare valves should be available, since they sometimes become blocked. A urine drainage bag may be used for draining a haemothorax.

Circulation

- Control external bleeding.
- Insert two large bore intravenous cannulae, which must be well secured. The limb must be splinted if movement is likely to occlude the cannula. Give crystalloid, colloid, or blood as appropriate, and take sufficient for the journey.
- Monitor urine output from an indwelling catheter.

Central nervous system

- Controlled ventilation is usually needed for head injured patients
- Give mannitol, or diuretics after discussion with the neurosurgeon
- Immobilize cervical, thoracic, and lumbar spine in suspected or confirmed spinal injuries

Fractures

- Apply appropriate splints and traction
- Consider a regional block as analgesia for fractures

Wounds

- Clean and dress wounds
- Give tetanus prophylaxis and antibiotics as required

The patient should be accompanied by a senior doctor. An anaesthetist must accompany patients with airway problems or who are intubated. Portable resuscitation equipment should be available throughout the journey. Treatment and monitoring must continue in transit. A pulse oximeter monitors pulse rate, oxygen saturation, and pulse volume. It may help in the early diagnosis of bleeding, airway, or ventilation problems. Analgesia should be given if the patient is conscious and in pain. Entonox may be used, but creates problems of bulk and supply on long journeys. Prolonged use may make the patient restless or confused. Incremental, low dose, intravenous morphine or diamorphine are probably the safest and most effective analgesics. Naloxone should be available to counteract any ventilatory depression. The effect of the chosen drug should always be assessed before transfer. Benzodiazepines should not be used if the patient is in pain, since they have no analgesic effect and they produce unpredictable sedation and may cause ventilatory depression. Patients who are intubated and ventilated should receive adequate intravenous sedation, analgesia, and a muscle relaxant. They should have a completely pain-free and amnesic journey. A record of events during transfer should be made. The receiving hospital must be given an expected time of arrival, so that appropriate preparations can be made.

Further reading

British Thoracic Society and others (1993). Guidelines for the management of asthma: a summary. *British Medical Journal*, **306**,776–82.

European Resuscitation Council (1996). *Resuscitation*, **31**, 187–230. Published by Elsevier Science Ireland, Ltd., Bay 15k, Shannon Industrial Estate, C. Clare, Ireland.

Hatch, D. J. (1985). Acute upper airway obstruction in children. In *Recent advances in anaesthesia and analgesia*, 15 (ed. R. S.

Atkinson and A. P. Adams), pp. 133–53. Churchill Livingstone, Edinburgh.
Langford, R. M. and Armstrong, R. F. (1989). Algorithm for managing injury from smoke inhalation. *British Medical Journal*, **299**, 902–5.

Part 2
Sedation

10 Sedation

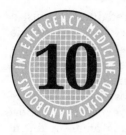

CHAPTER 10

10 Sedation

Key points in sedation

- The combination of sedation and analgesic drugs is potentially hazardous and should only be used by doctors trained in the management of unconscious patients.

- Monitoring and resuscitation equipment must be available when sedation is given.

- Patients who have received sedation should recover in a properly staffed and equipped area.

- It is unusual for severe agitation to respond to sedation alone. Before using drugs to calm such a patient a diagnosis should be made. Consider hypoxaemia, hypoglycaemia, urinary retention, or cerebral problems such as a head injury.

Scope and definition of sedation

Sedative drugs allay anxiety and hypnotic drugs produce sleep. Many drugs perform both functions at different doses. Commonly used drugs include benzodiazepines, chlormethiazole, phenothiazines, and butyrophenones. Intravenous anaesthetic induction agents may be used for sedation during minor procedures or to supplement local anaesthesia. Their use should be confined to anaesthetists who are able to deal with any airway compromise or ventilatory depression.

Oral sedatives may be used as pre-anaesthetic medication. In the A & E department, trauma may delay gastric emptying, and there may be insufficient time prior to surgery to allow adequate absorption of orally administered drugs. The use of certain premedicants may delay recovery from anaesthesia. However, premedication may be valuable in some situations. Anxious patients or children awaiting procedures may benefit from careful use of sedative medication.

Intravenous sedation usually involves the use of incremental doses of analgesic or sedative drugs to relieve anxiety, provide analgesia, and produce amnesia during brief, minor procedures. Sedatives are not analgesic and may produce restlessness or aggression in patients with pain. Simple sedation results in a calm, cooperative patient who can respond to verbal commands. Once verbal contact is lost, sedation has developed into general anaesthesia. Therefore intravenous sedation must only be performed by those competent to deal with an anaesthetized patient who may have lost protective laryngeal reflexes. Resuscitation equipment must be immediately available. Patients should fast before intravenous sedation. Adequately equipped, staffed recovery facilities are mandatory.

Pharmacology of sedative drugs

Benzodiazepines

Benzodiazepines have sedative, anxiolytic, anticonvulsant, and muscle-relaxant properties. The main sites of action of benzodiazepines are in the limbic and reticular activating systems of the brain. Benzodiazepine receptors have also been found in the spinal cord. Benzodiazepines act by facilitation of gamma aminobutyric acid (GABA), which is the principal inhibitory transmitter in the central nervous system. Chloride channels open in the presence of GABA, allowing chloride ions to pass into the neurone, causing hyperpolarization and decreased excitability.

Pharmacokinetics of benzodiazepines

Benzodiazepines have a large volume of distribution, because of their high lipid solubility. They are well absorbed from the gastrointestinal tract after oral or rectal administration. Enterohepatic recirculation may prolong their action. They are available for parenteral use. There is individual variation in dose requirement. Once absorbed, they are highly bound to plasma proteins, for example 96–98 per cent diazepam is bound to albumin; midazolam is less protein bound. Benzodiazepines cross the placenta easily, and can cause neonatal ventilatory depression, hypotonia, and hypothermia. Benzodiazepines are metabolized in the liver. Some metabolites have a prolonged effect, for example desmethyldiazepam (from diazepam and chlordiazepoxide) has a half life of 100 hours. Enzyme inhibition by drugs such as cimetidine can increase the effect of diazepam and midazolam. Elderly patients and those with liver failure may be sensitive to benzodiazepines because of reduced metabolism. Renal excretion is not important in the elimination of benzodiazepines. Renal failure does not usually lead to problems, except with oxazepam and lorazepam, which are excreted as water soluble glucuronides. Drugs with shorter half lives may be more suitable for use in the A & E department, especially if the patient is not to be admitted to hospital, for example temazepam or midazolam, rather than diazepam or lorazepam.

Diazepam
Diazepam is a basic drug with a pK_a of 3.4 so at phsiological pH it is 99.99 per cent unionized and poorly water soluble. It is presented for parenteral use as Diazemuls, a soya bean emulsion which will support the growth of bacteria and yeasts. Diazemuls cannot be used intramuscularly. The oral dose is 0.4–0.5 mg/kg in children and 10–20 mg in adults. If used intravenously, it should be titrated slowly every 2–3 minutes until the desired level of sedation is reached. The maximum dose in a healthy patient is 0.3 mg/kg, but prolonged sedation may result. Diazepam metabolism is not affected by hepatic blood flow but altered by variations in protein binding.

Temazepam
Temazepam is a metabolite of diazepam, which is well absorbed after oral administration, especially if the elixir is used rather than the gelatine capsules. It gives more rapid recovery than intravenous diazepam but less amnesia. The oral dose is 1 mg/kg in children and 20–40 mg in adults. Temazepam has its maximal effect one hour after adminis-

tration, in children it is indistingushable from placebo two hours after administration. The timing of administration is important, which may be a disadvantage in the A & E setting.

Midazolam

Midazolam is a drug whose water solubility is pH dependent. Below pH 4 it is water soluble, so the formulation is aqueous. At physiological pH its ring structure closes, giving it a pK_a of 6.2 and rendering it lipid soluble. It has a faster onset and produces more profound amnesia than diazepam. It has rapid clearance with no clinically important active metabolites. There is a subset of patients who metabolize midazolam more slowly than is usual. They may show prolonged effects after the drug. It can be used orally in children, at a dose of 0.5–0.75 mg/kg (fruit juice can be used to disguise the bitter taste). Intranasal and sublingual administration has been studied in children, but the former is unpleasant and the latter requires cooperation. Midazolam can be administered intramuscularly or intravenously. If given intravenously it must be titrated slowly to effect. Elderly patients can be quite sensitive to midazolam. The combination of midazolam with propofol is synergistic. The usual doses used for this combination are 0.04 mg/kg midazolam and 0.07 mg/kg propofol titrated to give the desired result. Midazolam metabolism is more dependent on liver blood flow and less affected by alterations in protein binding when compared to diazepam.

Lorazepam

Lorazepam is a longer acting benzodiazepine which can be given orally, intramuscularly, or intravenously. The usual oral dose in adults is 2–4 mg. It has no advantages in children and may lead to prolonged postoperative sedation. If it is used for intravenous sedation it has a slower onset and longer duration of action than diazepam. Its prolonged effect makes it unsuitable for use in the A & E department.

Indications for benzodiazepines
- Intravenous sedation during minor procedures
- Premedication prior to general anaesthesia
- Treatment of fits (e.g. epilepsy or local anaesthetic toxicity)

- Treatment of pre-eclampsia
- Reduction of muscle spasm during manipulation of dislocations
- Oral administration to reduce muscle spasm after trauma, for example in acute back pain

Contraindications to benzodiazepines
- The dose may be difficult to judge in very young or very frail patients
- Patients who have taken other sedatives, such as alcohol
- Patients with chest problems, who should never be sedated unless they are intubated and ventilated
- Patients in pain or very aggressive patients, who may become more aggressive after sedation
- Shocked patients, who may become hypotensive after benzodiazepines
- Head injured patients
- In porphyria temazepam is safe, lorazepam and midazolam may be safe, diazepam is contentious, and other benzodiazepines may be unsafe

Benzodiazepine antagonists

Flumazenil is a specific benzodiazepine antagonist. It has been used to treat benzodiazepine overdose or neonatal sedation. It has a short half life and the effect of the benzodiazepine may outlast that of the antagonist. It may cause fitting, cardiac arrhythmias, and acute withdrawal symptoms. It may be useful in establishing a diagnosis in patients with coma of unknown aetiology. It should not be used routinely to counteract benzodiazepine-induced sedation or to allow discharge of patients from hospital earlier than would otherwise be possible. The dose is 200 μg in adults given in small increments.

Chlormethiazole

Chlormethiazole is a sedative drug, related to vitamin B_1, which acts by affecting GABA transmission. It is given parenterally as a 0.8 per cent solution in 5 per cent dextrose, and may produce thrombophlebitis. The initial adult dose is

8–20 ml/min, and a maintenance dose of up to 1 litre every 12 hours may be required. It is 50 per cent bound to plasma protein and has an elimination half life of 3–5 hours. When given slowly it has a slow onset, producing sleep in 30–40 minutes. It has antiemetic effects. It is useful in the management of restlessness and agitation in elderly patients. It is spmetimes used for the treatment of alcohol withdrawal and pre-eclampsia. Care must be taken not to produce fluid overload when using this drug in patients with renal problems. It potentiates other sedative drugs, including general anaesthetics.

Phenothiazines

Phenothiazines are potent antipsychotic drugs that affect many different neurotransmitters at multiple sites in the nervous system. Phenothiazines with potent central anticholinergic effects are sedative, produce drying of secretions, and have antiemetic properties. They may produce dystonic reactions. The more sedative phenothiazines are used for premedication. Promethazine is well absorbed after oral administration in a dose of 0.5–1.0 mg/kg. It produces sedation within 30–40 minutes. It has a prolonged duration of action of up to 24 hours which limits its use in the A & E department. It may cause dizziness and disorientation in older patients. Trimeprazine is used for premedication in children. It is well absorbed after an oral dose of 2 mg/kg, and is available as a syrup. It may produce excitatory effects in some children. It produces better antiemesis than benzodiazepines, but has a more prolonged recovery. It should not be used in children under 2 years old.

Butyrophenones

Butyrophenones, are potent sedatives which act on many different neurotransmitters such as noradrenaline and dopamine. They have similar antipsychotic and antiemetic effects to phenothiazines, but are more likely to produce dystonic reactions and should not be used in children. Intravenous droperidol can be used with a strong opioid to produce intravenous sedation and 'neuroleptanalgesia' for minor procedures. Droperidol must never be given without opioid or sedative drugs, as unpleasant dysphoria is common. Hypotension may be produced. It is also used as an antiemetic, when a low dose of 1.25 mg is sufficient. It is used with opioids to reduce emesis during the use of patient-controlled analgesia (PCA). Even very low doses may result in dysphoria for up to 24 hours afterwards. It is not recommended for day cases.

Propofol (see p. 19)

Small increments of propofol may be used for sedation. Propofol has antiemetic properties. Its use should probably be confined to anaesthetists.

Combined sedation and analgesia

Combined sedation and analgesia is a popular but potentially hazardous technique. It should be used by non-anaesthetists only if they are adequately trained in airway management and resuscitation. A practical knowledge of drug dosage, effects, side-effects, and interactions is essential. The technique must be performed with full resuscitation equipment available. Monitoring similar to that used for general anaesthesia is required. Trained assistance for the person providing the sedation is mandatory. The person monitoring the patient should not be the same person who is performing the procedure. The patient must be fasted before sedation, as there is always the risk that airway control will be lost. Sedation is provided by an intravenous benzodiazepine, such as Diazemuls or midazolam. Analgesia is provided by Entonox or a parenteral opioid, such as morphine. Shorter acting opioids such as fentanyl or alfentanil may be useful. However, they may produce quite profound ventilatory depression. If the patient is likely to have pain after the procedure, postoperative pain relief may be needed sooner if short acting opioids have been used. The sedative effects of the benzodiazepine are potentiated by opioids or Entonox. Allowance must be made for any preoperative medication, such as intramuscular opioid. Sedation is also potentiated by alcohol and by medication such as antidepressants and antihistamines. The elderly are unpredictable in their response to sedatives, and may require minimal doses. Drugs should be titrated slowly intravenously. An opioid should be given in a dose to provide adequate analgesia, some sedation may also occur. Diazemuls or midazolam should then be titrated, using increments depending on the patient's size and age.

Patient controlled sedation has been used as a technique to provide optimal sedation during procedures. Devices similar to PCA machines are used, which have been modified to give a fast infusion with no lock-out (see p. 240). Propofol or midazolam have been used with this technique.

Verbal contact with the patient must be maintained during sedation. If verbal contact is lost simple sedation has progressed to general anaesthesia, and airway control may be compromised. The procedure may commence with the patient lightly sedated and pain free. Routine criteria for establishing recovery should be observed (see p. 94). This technique should not be used on children, because of the high risk of vomiting and aspiration, variability of response to the drugs, and the risk of limited cooperation.

Anaesthesia and analgesia for the reduction of common dislocations

The pain resulting from a dislocation is relieved by reduction of the joint. Early reduction limits the risk of associated joint or neurovascular problems. Analgesia may be required preoperatively. Immobilization using a sling or splint or supporting the limb on pillows provides some comfort so long as the limb remains immobile. Intramuscular diclofenac or ketoralac may be used, but some patients require an opioid. Patients requiring a general anaesthetic should be fasted; but occasionally neurovascular involvement necessitates an urgent reduction, in which case a rapid sequence induction technique must be used.

Dislocation of the shoulder

Patients vary greatly in their need for analgesia and anaesthesia for reduction of a dislocated shoulder. Muscle spasm of the periarticular muscles hinders reduction, but may be minimal in the elderly or if limb function has been affected by a cerebrovascular accident. There may be considerable resistance in large, muscular patients. It should not be assumed that a shoulder which suffers recurrent dislocation will necessarily be easy to reduce.

Various manoeuvres are used to reduce a dislocated shoulder; their success depends on a good technique supplemented by adequate analgesia and anaesthesia. It may be possible to reduce a shoulder without using a general anaesthetic; but if the patient is in pain attempts at reduction should be stopped immediately, and a general anaesthetic should be considered. Pain worsens muscle spasm and hinders reduction, as well as being unacceptable to the patient. Entonox alone may be sufficient in those with limited muscle mass, such as the elderly. The patient should receive a 3–4 minute 'top-up' of Entonox before the procedure is attempted. A combined sedation and analgesia technique may be used (see p. 219), but general anaesthesia is required if this is unsuccessful. Patients who have needed a general anaesthetic in the past may well require the same method for a recurrence of the problem.

Dislocation of the elbow

Urgent reduction is required when there is neurovascular involvement. This may be possible using Entonox, but an emergency general anaesthetic may be required. Brachial plexus block may be used for less urgent reductions.

Dislocation of the first metacarpophalangeal joint

This may be reduced using a combined radial and median nerve block. Occasionally open reduction is required, in which case a regional local anaesthetic technique or general anaesthetic may be used.

Dislocation of the finger

This commonly occurs on the sports field, and may be reduced at the time of injury without any analgesia. In the A & E department reduction may be performed using Entonox or a digital nerve block at the metacarpal level.

Dislocation of the patella

This can usually be reduced using Entonox.

Supplementing local anaesthesia

If local anaesthesia does not produce analgesia in the total area required and the block cannot be improved by administration of additional local anaesthetic, an alternative technique must be used. Surgery must never be commenced in the presence of inadequate local anaesthesia. It may sometimes be necessary to proceed to general anaesthesia. In some situations, particularly when the procedure is to be brief, it may be acceptable to supplement local anaesthesia with analgesic and/or sedative agents. Adjuvants must not be used to compensate for poor technique or failure to wait for local anaesthesia to take effect.

A variety of drugs and inhalational agents can be used to supplement local anaesthetic techniques. All of these are potent central nervous system depressants. The ventilatory depressant effects of benzodiazepines and opioids are additive if these drugs are used together. Therefore sedation using central nervous and ventilatory depressant drugs should only be practised by doctors able to manage an anaesthetized patient.

Patients who are selected for local anaesthesia because they are a poor risk for general anaesthesia should be given supplementary drugs with care. Any patient who has received adjuvant drugs must be kept in hospital for at least two hours afterwards, before being allowed home under the care of a responsible adult. Written instructions should be given about precautions to be taken and potential problems during the following 48 hours (see p. 96).

Indications for supplementation of local anaesthesia

- Adequate local anaesthesia achieved but the patient remains anxious.
- Adequate local anaesthesia but poor muscle relaxation.
- To increase patient comfort and allow the patient to remain still during tedious procedures such as wound toilet.
- To provide analgesia after the local anaesthetic has worn off. A longer acting local anaesthetic, such as bupivacaine may provide prolonged pain relief.

Contraindications to supplementation of local anaesthesia

- Airway obstruction.
- If local anaesthesia is totally inadequate.
- Serious cardiorespiratory, hepatic, or renal problems. Major endocrine or neuromuscular disorders may also lead to sensitivity to analgesics and sedatives.
- Head injury, depressed consciousness level, or intake of alcohol or sedative drugs.
- Children in whom intravenous supplementation is difficult to titrate.
- Elderly patients who may be very sensitive to analgesic or sedative drugs.

Techniques for supplementing local anaesthesia

- Entonox (see p. 23) can be a useful addition during local anaesthesia. It is a potent analgesic, which works quickly and wears off within minutes. It is probably the safest way to supplement local anaesthesia for a brief period.
- Benzodiazepines (see p. 214), such as Diazemuls or midazolam, are commonly used intravenously to produce sedation, anxiolysis, and muscle relaxation to supplement local blocks. They are not analgesics. They produce amnesia if given before the procedure. There is large individual variation in dose requirements for intravenous benzodiazepines. In adults midazolam should be given at the rate of 2 mg every 2 minutes to a maximum of 10 mg, and Diazemuls should be given at 2 mg every 2 minutes to a maximum of 20 mg. Midazolam has the advantage that it produces a less prolonged effect than Diazemuls.
- Opioids (see p. 242) can be used to provide additional intra- and postoperative pain relief. Morphine should be given slowly after being diluted so that the minimum dose necessary is used, for example 2 mg intravenously every 2 minutes up to a maximum of 10 mg in an adult. Alfentanil and fentanyl may be useful in this situation. These drugs must be diluted and titrated slowly due to their ventilatory depressant effect. Naloxone should be immediately available.

- Propofol can be used in small doses to supplement local anaesthesia. Its use should be confined to anaesthetists as it is easy to progress from sedation to general anaesthesia using this agent.

The severely agitated patient in the A & E department

The agitated patient poses a challenge to nursing and medical skills. Patients may become violent following alcohol or drug abuse and are at risk of hurting themselves or others. They may be unable to give a history and so reliance must be placed on accompanying paramedics, relatives, or friends. Check whether the patient is carrying any drugs or has a 'MedicAlert' disc. A thorough examination must be made despite the difficult circumstances, since multiple pathology may exist. For example, agitation in a known alcoholic should not be assumed to be due to alcohol intoxication until other common causes such as head injury have been excluded. The blood glucose should be checked, initially by stick test.

Common causes of an agitated patient seen in an A & E department include

- alcohol abuse
- drug overdose
- drug abuse
- solvent abuse
- hypoglycaemia
- post-ictal states
- head injury
- hypoxaemia
- hysteria
- acute psychosis
- pain
- urinary retention
- electrolyte imbalance

Agitation should settle once the cause is treated. Sedation should rarely be required. It should be considered if there is a serious risk of injury to the patient or if aggressive behaviour prevents urgent treatment. Patients with acute asthma attack, airway obstuction, head injury, chest trauma, or ventilatory failure should not be sedated.

The basic resuscitation principles of 'Airway, Breathing, Circulation' should be followed.

Analgesia may be given, when necessary, once resuscitation is complete. Persistent agitation in a head injured patient requires neurosurgical referral.

Intravenous Diazemuls may be carefully titrated in agitated patients following a drug overdose or an epileptic fit. Resuscitation equipment must be immediately available in case ventilation is depressed. Agitation due to alcohol or drug withdrawal may also be treated with Diazemuls. Chlormethiazole is an alternative for managing alcohol withdrawal. This may be given intravenously for delirium tremens or severe agitation. Oral chlormethiazole or chlordiazepoxide may be prescribed for less severe withdrawal symptoms. Acute psychosis may be treated with haloperidol 1.5–20.0 mg orally daily in divided doses. In severe cases 2–10 mg (increasing to 30 mg for emergency control) intramuscular haloperidol may be used. Half the adult dose should be used in elderly or debilitated patients.

Further reading

Drug and Therapeutics Bulletin (1991). Management of behavioural emergencies. *Drug and Therapeutics Bulletin*, **29**, 62–4.

O'Boyle, C. A., Harris, D., and Barry, H. (1987). Comparison of oral midazolam and intravenous diazepam in outpatient oral surgery. *British Joournal of Anaesthesia*, **59**, 746–54.

Ullyot, S. C. (1992). Paediatric premedication. *Canadian anaesthetists society Journal*, **39**, 533–6.

White, P .F., Vasconez, L. O., Matnes, S. A., Way, W. L., and Wender, L.A. (1988). Comparison of midazolam and diazepam for sedation during plastic surgery. *Plastic and Reconstructive surgery*, **81**, 703–10.

Part 3
Analgesia

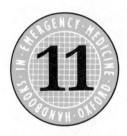

CHAPTER 11

Analgesia

Key points in analgesia

- Local anaesthesia is a valuable adjunct in certain injuries. Care must be taken not to mask important physical signs such as those of compartment syndrome.

- Analgesics must be administered intravenously in small increments until the required response is obtained. Opioids and non-steroidal anti-inflammatory drugs are effective analgesics which can be given parenterally. Antiemetics may be needed in some patients.

- Entonox is a useful rapid acting agent for brief procedures.

- Paediatric doses of analgesic drugs should be calculated using the weight of the child.

- Patients with acute abdominal pain should receive pain relief early. This does not interfere with physical signs and may make diagnosis easier.

- Care must be taken when using analgesics in head injured patients, opioids may further depress consciousness.

Pain control in the A & E department

At least three-quarters of new patients attending the A & E department are likely to have some degree of pain. In practical terms, a department with 70 000 new patients a year will see over 50 000 patients with pain.

Patients vary in their response to pain and the need for analgesia. Personality, ethnic origin, environment, and previous experiences all influence the reaction to pain. Some patients refuse analgesia, or never collect prescriptions for analgesics. Some patients demand immediate analgesia, while others still expect to be in pain when they have left the department. Patients may present with the typical acute pain of myocardial ischaemia or the chronic pain of lower back problems. The pain may form part of an intricate web of personal, family, social, or other problems, and a single specific cause may be difficult to elucidate.

The severity of the pain cannot be judged by the appearance of the injury – for example, severe facial injuries can be remarkably pain free, and there is sometimes a period of relative analgesia in severely crushed fingers before they become very painful. However, an innocuous looking subungual haematoma or a deeply situated abscess can be excruciatingly painful.

Pain prevention

Pain prevention is an important part of the A & E department's practise. Care must be taken to ensure that nursing and medical procedures cause the least possible discomfort to the patient. Health education, particularly regarding accident prevention and first aid techniques, should also be available to patients.

Methods of pain relief

Many factors are involved when choosing the best method of pain relief. The patient's age, size, and personality, and preexisting medical conditions or medication should be considered. The cause, severity, and nature of the pain are important. Plans to admit to hospital or operate may affect the choice of analgesic.

Explanation

Patients require a clear explanation of the diagnosis, the treatment, and the expected time to recovery. A clear understanding will reduce the number of unnecessary visits caused by patients expecting too much too soon. Pain is easier to manage when the patient understands the problem and can anticipate the outcome.

Splintage
Immobilization of fractures or dislocations often provides adequate analgesia, although pain may persist until reduction has been performed. Entonox may be used during application of the splint. Severe pain continuing after splintage should raise the question of some possible associated problem, such as neurovascular damage or the plaster or dressing being too tight.

Dressings
Pain due to minor burns or finger-tip injuries often settles once an appropriate dressing is applied.

Definitive treatment
Trephining a nail with a tense subungual haematoma or reducing a dislocated joint often gives immediate pain relief.

Local anaesthesia
Local anaesthesia can be a valuable technique for providing analgesia for certain injuries. Side effects such as vomiting or ventilatory depression, which can occur with opioids, are not a problem with local anaesthesia. It does not affect consciousness level, which is useful when dealing with a head injured patient. Good analgesia can aid subsequent examination. A nerve block may be used after initial assessment and emergency treatment have been given. The neurological status of the area to be anaesthetized must always be recorded before the block is performed. Once analgesia is established a more thorough examination may be possible – wounds can be explored, and the patient will be more ready to test movement, for example in a crushed finger. Following local blockade, fractures, such as a fractured shaft of the femur, may be splinted. The patient should then have a pain-free passage through the radiology department. Definitive treatment may also be possible under the original nerve block. Nerve blocks are discussed in Part 4 (Page 271).

Oral analgesics
Oral analgesics are commonly prescribed in the A & E department. The therapeutic effect varies little among the various drugs used for mild to moderate pain, and drug choice should be based on the incidence of side effects and

cost (Yates *et al.* 1984). Hospital purchasing policy may dictate what is available. Current medication must be reviewed before prescribing analgesics, as some patients are already taking analgesics, or have a suitable supply at home. A history of allergy or peptic ulceration should be sought and recorded. Instructions for the use of analgesics must be clearly explained and written down if necessary. It is advisable to use just a few analgesics, and to become familiar with their dosage, side-effects, drug interactions, and expected responses. Paracetamol may be used for mild pain. Moderate pain or the pain of musculoskeletal or bony problems may be controlled by paracetamol and dihydrocodeine combinations. A non-steroidal anti-inflammatory drug may be useful for acute arthritis, soft tissue injuries, bone and joint injuries, or dental pain. More severe pain may be helped by stronger drugs such as tramadol. The type, dose, and amount of drug prescribed should be recorded clearly on the A & E card.

Parenteral analgesics

Opioids are the most commonly used parenteral analgesics. The intravenous route is preferable, providing a predictable and rapid onset of action. Peak plasma concentrations are rapidly attained, enabling easy assessment of need and appropriate titration of the drug. A decline in the initial peak concentration limits the time during which a toxic reaction may occur. The intramuscular route is much less predictable, with altered perfusion producing erratic absorption and ineffective analgesia. This route should not be used in patients with a low cardiac output. The intramuscular route may be used in children who need strong analgesia, but do not require intravenous therapy – for example when dressing superficial burns.

Morphine is a commonly used opioid. Opioids may cause vomiting, which can be controlled by prochlorperazine or cyclizine. Morphine should be given in a dose which relieves the pain, which may be 3 mg for a frail elderly patient or 20 mg for a fit young adult. It should be diluted to 1 mg/ml with normal saline, and given incrementally. The syringe must be labelled clearly. Half the calculated dose may be given by slow intravenous injection. This may be followed by 1.0 mg increments until analgesia is obtained. A smaller initial dose should be used in elderly or shocked patients. Other opioid analgesics such as diamorphine may be used.

The non-steroidal anti-inflammatory drugs diclofenac and ketorolac are effective in the treatment of a variety of painful conditions. Absence of neurological effects makes them valuable for use in head injured patients. Great care must be taken in patients with renal failure, as this may be made much worse. These drugs are contraindicated in patients with a history of asthma, peptic ulcers or colitis. (see p. 250).

Entonox

Entonox is a 50 per cent mixture of oxygen and nitrous oxide. Its physical properties and pharmacology are discussed on p. 23. Entonox may be given by a patient demand valve that can be overridden. A similar mixture may be delivered from an anaesthetic machine using a Laerdal resuscitation bag or anaesthetic circuit.

Entonox provides 50 per cent oxygen but this may not be sufficient for some hypoxaemic patients. Analgesia occurs after about 45 seconds and quickly subsides once the drug is withdrawn. There should be no drop in blood pressure or consciousness level, although prolonged use may cause confusion and restlessness. The high oxygen concentration may, in theory, depress ventilation in patients dependent on hypoxic drive. In practice this is not usually a problem. The efficacy of Entonox depends upon good patient compliance. Those unable to use the apparatus should be given another form of analgesia.

Entonox may be administered by the patient or attendant. The patient should be warned that he or she may feel dizzy or become drowsy. The mask should form a comfortable and complete seal around the nose and mouth, and the patient should take deep breaths until analgesia is obtained. Facial injuries may prevent the use of this apparatus. Those who dislike or cannot use masks may use a mouthpiece. An assistant may need to hold the mask if the patient has upper-limb injuries or gets tired. If the pain returns more Entonox may be given.

Nitrous oxide rapidly diffuses into air-filled spaces, causing expansion of air in the pleural cavity, the bowel, the middle ear, the cranial cavity, and air emboli. Entonox should never be used in patients with decompression sickness (caisson disease) or compound skull fractures. It is best avoided in patients with bowel obstruction. A pneumothorax should be drained before Entonox is used.

Entonox may be used for minor procedures, such as the application of splints or the reduction of a dislocated finger or patella. A dislocated shoulder may be successfully reduced under Entonox, but in many cases it is insufficient to overcome the associated muscle spasm. Supplementary analgesia may be required, or a different anaesthetic technique may be used. Entonox can prove a useful supplement to an incomplete nerve block. A grossly deficient nerve block should not be supplemented by Entonox, but should be repeated or abandoned.

A general plan for the management of severe pain

Ensure that the patient has received adequate resuscitation and is well oxygenated. Hypoxaemia can mimic some signs of pain and make the patient restless. Check that there is no immediately remediable cause for the pain, such as a distended bladder that needs catheterizing or a splint that needs adjusting. Administer 50 per cent nitrous oxide and oxygen. If analgesia is inadequate give incremental intravenous doses of an opioid, such as morphine, up to 0.2 mg/kg. If pain persists ensure that naloxone is available; be prepared to support ventilation, and give further increments of morphine. If analgesia is adequate, but it becomes apparent that agitation and anxiety are the problems, consider the incremental intravenous use of 5.0 to 10.0 mg Diazemuls or 2.5 to 5.0 mg midazolam. Doctors with limited airway skills should be careful about combinig opioids and benzodiazepines in view of the risk of ventilatory depression.

Pain theories and general considerations

In 1644 Descartes suggested that pain was produced by stimulation of specific receptors which relayed messages to the brain via nerves. The idea that pain was mediated by specific pathways was replaced by the pattern theory, which suggested that pain could be produced by all nerves, and depended upon generation of a pattern of impulses rather than on anatomical considerations. The 'gate theory' of pain modulation at a spinal level was proposed by Melzack and Wall. An understanding of central modulation, descending inhibition, and the involvement of neurotransmitters has further clarified pain mechanisms.

In 1968 Mountcastle defined pain as 'that sensory experience evoked by stimuli that injure'. Progress in the understanding of pain can be seen by a change in definition in 1979, when Merskey defined pain as 'an unpleasant sensory and emotional experience associated with actual or potential tissue damage, or described in terms of such damage'. This definition emphasizes the importance of the emotional aspects of pain.

Pain is a complex experience, which involves sensory, affective, and cognitive components that manifest as a pattern of behaviour with social consequences. Pain is the commonest reason for patients to seek medical advice, and patients should always be believed when they complain of pain. The best definition of pain is 'what the patient says hurts'.

'Pain threshold' refers to the least experience of pain which the patient can recognize, and is fairly constant for each person. 'Pain tolerance' is the greatest level of pain which the patient is prepared to endure, and may vary in different situations. If a patient is complaining of what seems to be an excessive amount of pain for a given situation, it is not a 'low pain threshold' which is the problem, but a lack of ability to tolerate that pain in that situation. Such a patient should be treated with sympathy.

Sensory aspects

A stimulus usually causes pain by the activation of nociceptors, which are terminals of myelinated and unmyelinated nerve fibres that are abundant in skin and musculoskeletal tissues. The afferent fibres of nociception are either thin myelinated A delta fibres (conduction velocity 10–20 m/s) or slow unmyelinated C fibres (conduction velocity 1 m/s). Cutaneous A delta fibres subserve immediate, sharp, easily localized pain. C fibres give rise to slower, burning, more diffuse pain. Visceral pain is transmitted by A delta, C, vagal, and sympathetic nerve fibres. It is difficult to localize, and is often referred to other structures – for example, splenic pain is referred to the shoulder tip.

The A delta and C fibres enter the spinal cord via the lateral division of the dorsal root, and give off ascending branches which terminate in the dorsal horn. There are two main types of projection from this level:

- nociceptive specific neurones, which respond to high intensity stimulation
- wide dynamic range neurones, which respond to light touch from the periphery of the receptive field and high intensity stimulation from the centre of the receptive field

The nociceptive afferents have connections with motor and sympathetic fibres, and nociceptive impulses may therefore also cause muscle spasm and vasoconstriction. The ascending nociceptive paths terminate at several thalamic nuclei, which in turn project to the cerebral cortex. There are also connections within the limbic and reticular systems.

Nociceptive transmission is subject to modulation at several different sites. At a segmental level there is 'gating' of nociceptive impulses in the substantia gelatinosa of the spinal cord. Large diameter A beta fibres transmitting signals from low threshold afferents, for example touch, pressure, and vibration, inhibit transmission of information in nociceptive paths. This is the underlying principle for analgesia during manipulation, massage, and transcutaneous nerve stimulation. A mechanism similar to 'gate control' operates at a higher level to exert central control on nociception. This is manifest when patients in intense emotional situations do not seem to feel pain – for example, men in battle.

Affective aspects

Emotion and mood have a very important role in the pain experience. In acute pain the patient is fearful and often has negative expectations, which are exacerbated by uncertainty. Depression is common in patients with chronic pain conditions, who may have had years of unremitting pain. Appreciation of the patients' fears and empathic support are vital when dealing with patients in pain.

Cognitive aspects

Patients try to rationalize the causes and likely outcomes of pain, and this element of the pain experience may alter their pain tolerance. Previous occurrences, inappropriate beliefs, and a lack of control over the outcome all act to worsen the pain. Patients from different cultures express pain differently. Sympathetic explanation and realistic reassurance are important in providing good pain relief.

Pharmacology of analgesics

An analgesic drug relieves pain non-specifically in a dose which does not impair consciousness. Some drugs alleviate pain by a direct effect on the cause, for example angina is relieved by the action of glyceryl trinitrate on coronary vessels, but these drugs are not designated analgesics. Anaesthetic gases and vapours may also be analgesic (see p. 20).

Opioids

Opioids are useful in the treatment of dull pain, mediated by C fibres. They are less effective for sharp pain, which is carried by A delta fibres. Opioids often only partly relieve dysaesthetic pain caused by nerve damage, such as postherpetic neuralgia or brachial plexus injury.

Classification

The term opioid includes all naturally occurring and synthetic drugs, which bind to opioid receptors and exert an effect. The term opiate is reserved for drugs that are structurally related to opium alkaloids. Some opioid drugs also have features that are inconsistent with this classification, such as meptazinol and tramadol, since only a proportion of their effect is mediated via opioid receptors. Opioid are classified according to their actions at different receptors. The μ, K, and δ receptors are associated with analgesia. The σ receptor is not a true opioid receptor and is associated with dysphoria. Although opioid analgesia is mainly mediated by central nervous effects, opioids also produce analgesia by actions on the spinal cord and peripheral nerves. Opioids have been used intrathecally and epidurally.

Drugs can be classified according to their affinity for receptors and their efficacy once bound. An agonist binds to a receptor and exerts an effect which increases with increasing dose; morphine is a μ agonist. Agonists may have different efficacies, for example morphine is more efficacious than codeine, but both bind to the μ site. A partial agonist binds to a receptor and exerts an effect, which increases with increasing dose until it reaches a plateau, for example, buprenorphine is a partial μ agonist. An antagonist binds to a receptor and has no effect, for example, naloxone is a μ antagonist. Some drugs act as agonists at one receptor and antagonists on a different population of receptors (agonist–antagonists), for example, nalbuphine is a partial agonist at K receptors and an antagonist at μ sites. Partial agonists and agonist–antagonists are not very useful in the treatment of severe pain, because of the ceiling effect, for example, the use of more than 30 mg of nalbuphine does not produce an increase in analgesia. Efficacy determines the clinical situations in which different opioids should be chosen. Inappropriate use of weak analgesics leads to inadequate relief, for example, codeine is not efficacious enough to be used for severe pain.

Physico-chemical properties

The physico-chemical properties of opioids (Table 11.1) affect their activity. The ability of a drug to diffuse through membranes to receptors depends upon its lipid solubility and the relative concentrations of ionized and unionized forms. All opioids are bases, with different pK_a values. Alfentanil is a weak base (pK_a 6.5), which is 89 per cent unionized at pH 7.4; methadone is a strong base (pK_a 9.3), which is 1 per cent unionized at physiological pH. Alfentanil is therefore more freely diffusable than methadone. All opioids are protein bound. The unionized, unbound fraction is the diffusible fraction. The greater this is the more quickly the drug will diffuse into tissues. Morphine has a high diffusibility but a slow onset because of its poor lipid solubility. Diamorphine and alfentanil are diffusible and lipid soluble and so act quickly.

Table 11.1 • Physico-chemical properties of opiods

	pK_a	Unionized fraction (%)	Diffusible fraction (%)
Morphine	7.9	23	16
Diamorphine	7.6	37	22
Pethidine	8.5	7	2
Fentanyl	8.4	9	1.7
Alfentanil	6.5	89	8
Methadone	9.3	1	0.1
Buprenorphine	8.4	9	0.4

Routes of administration, metabolism, and elimination

Patients must be treated as individuals whose perceptions of pain and analgesic needs differ. Analgesics should be titrated to each patient's response. There is large individual variation in dose requirements, which is increased by differences in drug absorption. Less lipid soluble opioids, such as morphine, are poorly absorbed from the gut, and are subject to hepatic 'first pass' metabolism. The oral:parenteral dose requirement for morphine is at least 5:1 after a single oral dose. Highly lipid soluble drugs such as pethidine and diamorphine are more readily absorbed following oral administration. Oral morphine is not effective in acute pain, but is useful in chronic pain, where long term administration allows a constant plasma level to be sustained. Sublingual administration of opioids, such as buprenorphine, reduces 'first pass' metabolism, but the drug must be very lipid soluble and potent to be given by this route. Rectal administration produces good absorption, for example, oxycodone, but there is large variation within and between subjects. Absorption is sometimes quite slow following intramuscular opioids, for example, peak analgesia is not achieved until 60 minutes after intramuscular morphine. Lipid soluble drugs such as diamorphine are well absorbed after subcutaneous administration, this route is used for diamorphine infusion in cancer pain. It is not appropriate to use the oral, sublingual, rectal, intramuscular, or subcutaneous routes for administration of opioids for severe, acute pain.

Opioids should be given intravenously if an immediate effect is needed. Peak analgesia occurs 10–20 minutes after the administration of intravenous morphine. A fourfold difference in plasma minimum effective analgesic concentration (MEAC) after intravenous opioid administration reflects individual differences in drug requirements. In order to sustain stable plasma concentrations it is logical to give opioids as an intravenous infusion, rather than as intermittent boluses. The infusion must be preceded by a loading dose to achieve MEAC, which would otherwise take 4–6 times the elimination half-life of the drug. Fewer side effects occur if the loading dose is given as a fast infusion, rather than as a bolus. The disadvantage of a continuous opioid infusion is that it is not titrated to the patient's needs. Continuous infusions for acute pain also require careful patient monitoring which may not be practical in the A & E setting. Patient controlled analgesia (PCA) systems allow the patient to regulate their own pain relief using a pump which delivers a dose of intravenous opioid on demand. The patient must be rendered pain free with intravenous opioid before being connected to the PCA machine, otherwise they will not be able to achieve analgesia. Background infusion is unnecessary in adults and may increase the likelihood of adverse effects. A PCA device is safer than a continuous infusion of opioid as the patient titrates the dose and does not administer opioid when there is no pain. The bolus and the time during which no further demands will be met ('lock-out') can all be varied, a typical setting for morphine would allow a 1–1.5 mg bolus and a 5 minute lock-out time. The introduction of PCA machines into the A & E department requires careful staff training.

Adverse effects
Pain is the physiological antagonist of many of the adverse effects of opioids. Ventilatory depression is seen in subjects without pain who take opioids; but large doses can be safely given to patients with severe pain. The incidence of side effects is dose related, and is similar with all opioids if equianalgesic doses are used. Sedation often occurs after opioid administration, and can be profound in opioid overdose in which painful stimuli are not present. If opioids are taken by subjects without pain, psychological and physical dependence occur. There is tolerance, with increasing dose

requirements and drug-seeking behaviour. Withdrawal of the drug results in psychological and physical signs and symptoms. If opioids are given to patients with acute pain these problems do not occur. Therefore there is no need to withhold opioids from patients in pain because of fears about addiction. Patients who are used to large doses of opioids, such as those with cancer or addicts who then develop acute pain often need high doses of analgesics to relieve their pain.

Opioids cause miosis. As opioids are bases, they may cause histamine release. The cardiovascular effects of opioids are minimal. Large doses may cause bradycardia and vasodilatation sufficient to produce hypotension. Reduction in pain after opioid administration, especially following myocardial infarction, may improve cardiovascular status. Centrally mediated ventilatory depression occurs after opioid administration, with a reduction in minute ventilation and a decreased response to the ventilatory stimulant effect of carbon dioxide. Opioid overdose kills patients by depressing breathing. Partial agonists have a ceiling effect for ventilatory depression, as well as for analgesia.

Nausea and vomiting following opioids are caused by stimulation of the chemoreceptor trigger zone, and are worse in ambulant patients. Opioid induced emesis should be treated by drugs acting centrally, such as phenothiazines, rather than by those acting peripherally, such as metoclopramide. Patients on long term opioids tend to develop tolerance to nausea, and often only require short term treatment with antiemetics. Gastric emptying and propulsive activity in the gut are reduced by opioids. A patient who has received opioids prior to general anaesthesia should be treated as having a full stomach. Metoclopramide may be administered in this situation to try to reduce the risk of aspiration of gastric contents, but its effect is not guaranteed. Smooth muscle tone is increased by opioids. Biliary and ureteric spasm occurs after most opioids, even pethidine. Retention of urine may occur after opioid administration. Uterine contractions are not affected by opioids. Opioids cross the placenta readily, and should be used with care in labouring women, as they affect the neonate, whose metabolic elimination processes are under developed.

Contraindications
- Ventilatory depression (less than 10 breaths/minute). Carefully titrated pain control may improve ventilatory function following rib fractures or in patients with underlying chest disease whose breathing is compromised by pain or trauma.
- Status asthmaticus in an unventilated patient.
- Raised intracranial pressure (ICP) sufficient to impair consciousness level in an unventilated patient. The careful use of opioids may help to reduce ICP in patients with multiple injuries who are severely hypertensive because of pain. However, adequate ventilation must be maintained.
- Patients taking monoamine oxidase inhibitors should not receive pethidine or its derivatives.
- Opioids should be used with caution in the presence of other CNS depressants and in patients with hypopituitarism, hypothyroidism, or chest, renal, or hepatic impairment.

Opioid toxicity
Opioid overdose is manifest by sedation, ventilatory depression, and miosis. It should be treated by standard resuscitation and intravenous naloxone (adult 5–6 μg/kg, neonate 5–10 μg/kg). Naloxone is a competitive opioid antagonist with a duration of action of 15–20 minutes. An intramuscular injection (adult 800 μg, neonate 200 μg) or an intravenous infusion may be necessary. Patients who have had significant ventilatory depression following opioids must be carefully monitored following recovery, as relapse is possible. Naloxone should be avoided in patients who have been given opioids for pain, unless they are at serious risk from ventilatory depression. The sudden reversal of analgesia may cause profound cardiovascular effects, such as arrhythmias and hypertension. Naloxone is relatively contraindicated in opioid addicts, as acute opioid withdrawal will occur.

Strong opioids
Morphine is the standard strong opioid against which all others are compared. Its large diffusible fraction compen-

sates for its poor lipid solubility. It produces analgesia without impairing consciousness, although some patients may become drowsy, especially after the first dose. The parenteral dose is 0.1–0.2 mg/kg. It should be given intravenously in the A & E setting. Its absorption after intramuscular injection is very variable, the peak effect may occur anything between 4 and 60 minutes after injection. Its duration of effect is 3–5 hours. Therefore it must be given at least every 4 hours to achieve pain control or via a PCA device. It is metabolized by the liver to morphine-3-glucuronide and morphine-6-glucuronide, which may accumulate in the presence of renal failure and lead to prolonged sedation.

Diamorphine is a semisynthetic opioid which is much more lipid soluble than morphine. It is the prodrug of morphine. It is rapidly hydrolysed in the blood and liver to 6-acetyl morphine and morphine, both of which are responsible for its analgesic effect. Diamorphine is better absorbed after oral administration. It has a more rapid effect than morphine when given parenterally, when it has twice the potency of morphine. It is much more water soluble and can be given as a very small volume intramuscular injection (100 mg will dissolve in 0.2 ml water) or as a subcutaneous infusion, where it is very useful in palliative care.

Pethidine is a synthetic drug which is structurally similar to atropine. The parenteral dose is 1 mg/kg. It is more lipid soluble and more protein bound than morphine. Its diffusible fraction is low which offsets the effect of its greater lipid solubility. It is absorbed orally (oral: parenteral dose 3:1). Its duration of action is only 2–3 hours. Its side-effects are similar to those of morphine if equianalgesic doses are compared. It has no advantages in the treatment of biliary or renal colic. It is metabolized to norpethidine, which may accumulate in renal failure and cause convulsions.

Fentanyl is a synthetic opioid which is mainly used during anaesthesia. It has high lipophilicity and protein binding, but a small diffusible fraction. It has a large apparent volume of distribution because of its high lipid solubility and its red cell and tissue binding. It has a rapid onset and brief duration of action. There are secondary peaks in plasma concentration after its administration.

Alfentanil is a synthetic opioid which has quite different pharmacokinetics. It has the lowest pK_a of all the opioids and therefore is highly unionized in plasma. This gives it much higher diffusibility than fentanyl. It has a very rapid onset and brief duration of effect following a single dose. It has a smaller volume of distribution than fentanyl and a shorter half life. It is useful during day-case anaesthesia.

Remifentanil is a new synthetic opioid which is metabolized by plasma esterases. It is used as a bolus of 1.0 μg/kg or an infusion of 0.1μg/kg/min. Its effect wears off rapidly and therefore it has a wide safety margin. It is safe in patients with hepatic and renal problems. It has no clinically important metabolites. It may be useful in the management of head injuries. Its rapid offset means that postoperative analgesia is needed immediately.

Methadone is a synthetic opioid which is well absorbed by the oral route. It has a slow clearance. It is therefore difficult to titrate and not recommended. It has been used to try to wean addicts from other strong opioids, but produces a dependence of its own. It may accumulate in elderly patients and those with renal failure.

Buprenorphine is a semisynthetic partial agonist at the μ site and an antagonist at the K site. It is well absorbed by the sublingual and parenteral routes, and has a long duration of action because of its high receptor affinity. The dose is 3–5 μg/kg. The incidence of side effects is similar to those of morphine. It has a ceiling effect for analgesia and ventilatory depression, but it may be difficult to reverse because of its strong receptor binding.

Nalbuphine is a synthetic partial K agonist and μ antagonist. The dose is 0.15 mg/kg. There is no further increase in analgesia when more than 30 mg is given to an adult. It does not have the same analgesic potential as morphine. There is an incidence of psychomimetic effects.

Tramadol is a synthetic opioid which also has non-opioid analgesic actions via central inhibition of noradrenaline reuptake and facilitation of 5-hydroxytryptamine release. About 30 per cent of the effect of tramadol is reversible by naloxone. It is useful in the A & E setting for moderate to severe pain. It is not recommended for children under 12 years. Tramadol may be given by the oral, intramuscular or intravenous route. It has about one-fifth to one-tenth the potency of morphine, the usual dose is 50–100 mg every 4–6 hours. It may lead to emesis in 30–35 per cent of patients. It is less likely to cause ventilatory depression than most other opioids. It is metabolized to an active compound o-desmethyltramadol, but this is not clinically important. Its effects may be prolonged in patients with renal or hepatic impairment. It has been associated with convulsions when used in conjunction with tricyclic antidepressants.

Weak opioids

Codeine is a natural alkaloid, methyl morphine. It is more lipid soluble than morphine and better absorbed orally. The dose is 30–60 mg 4-hourly. The small dose (8–10 mg) found in some proprietary combination analgesics probably has little effect. It is available as a fixed combination with paracetamol (paracetamol 500 mg/codeine 30 mg) which is more effective for moderate pain. It causes constipation. Codeine is 10–20 per cent metabolized to morphine, which contributes to its analgesic action.

Dihydrocodeine is a semisynthetic derivative of codeine which is a better analgesic. It is well absorbed orally, and the dose is 30–60 mg 4-hourly. A slow release preparation is available. Children and elderly patients may suffer from side-effects such as confusion and disorientation.

Dextropropoxyphene is a mild analgesic, of similar potency to codeine, which is often combined with 500 mg paracetamol in a dose of 65 mg (co-proxamol). This combination should perhaps be avoided, as in overdose it may produce profound ventilatory depression, and is a common cause of death.

Meptazinol is a synthetic opioid similar in structure to pethidine, but not all its analgesic effect is mediated via opioid receptors. The dose is 1–1.5 mg/kg parenterally or 2–3 mg/kg orally. It is used as an alternative to codeine for moderate pain.

Simple analgesics and non-steroidal anti-inflammatory drugs (NSAIDs)

Paracetamol is a simple analgesic without anti-inflammatory actions. Many other drugs with antipyretic and anti-inflammatory properties are analgesics. Most of these drugs are analgesic in single dose, and only have anti-inflammatory actions after repeated administration. They are used for musculoskeletal pain, when they reduce swelling, joint stiffness, and muscle tenderness, but do not influence the progression of diseases. They are valuable in treatment of somatic pain such as that following trauma or surgery. NSAIDs may decrease opioid requirements. They are effective in the treatment of visceral pain such as renal colic and dysmenorrhea. They are routinely used in the palliation of cancer pain especially in patients with bone metastases. Paracetamol is the most common simple analgesic given to children. NSAIDs can be used in those over one year of age, for example diclofenac and ibuprofen.

Mode of action

Although prostaglandins do not produce pain, they sensitize peripheral nerve endings to other agents, such as histamine or bradykinin. Most NSAIDs modulate the effect of peripheral chemical pain mediators by inhibiting cyclo-oxygenase, which reduces prostaglandin synthesis (Table 11.2). Some analgesic and antipyretic effects of NSAIDs and paracetamol are due to inhibition of cyclo-oxygenase in the central nervous system. Analgesic and anti-inflammatory activity does not depend solely on reduction of prostaglandin synthesis. Aspirin is as potent as paracetamol, but the latter only has one-tenth of the capacity of the former to inhibit cyclo-oxygenase. NSAIDs also reduce superoxide generation, scavenge free radicals, reduce inhibitory cell migration, and stabilize lysosomal membranes.

Pharmacokinetics

NSAIDs have many chemical structures with different potencies and duration of action (Table 11.3). Some are pro-drugs, such as sulindac and fenbufen. Most are rapidly absorbed after oral or rectal administration, and some are available parenterally. Topical preparations may be useful in treatment of acute muscular and ligamentous problems. NSAIDs are weak acids and most have pK_a values of 3–6. They are all more than 90 per cent protein bound. Their acid nature means that, at physiological pH, NSAIDs are mainly in the ionized form, which is not freely diffusible. In acid environments such as the stomach, the kidney, and inflamed joints, the amount of unionized NSAID increases. Synovial half life in diseased joints is often extended compared to

Table 11.2 • Action of non-steroidal anti-inflammatory drugs

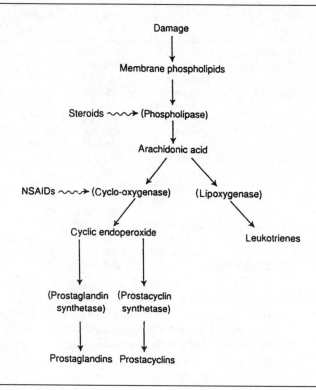

plasma half life, which may explain the prolonged effect of NSAIDs seen clinically. Most NSAIDs are metabolized in the liver, with inactive products excreted renally. NSAIDs interact with many other drugs. They may increase the effect of lithium, warfarin, and ACE inhibitors. They may reduce the effect of diuretics and antihypertensive agents.

Classification
Paracetamol is not an anti-inflammatory drug, but it is a centrally acting analgesic and antipyretic. It is rapidly absorbed from the small gut, producing analgesia in 30–40 minutes which lasts four hours. It lacks gastric side effects because it does not inhibit peripheral prostaglandin synthesis. The adult dose is 1 g up to four times daily. It is sometimes used in fixed combination with weak opioids such as codeine and dextropropoxyphene. In children the oral dose is 10–15

Table 11.3 • Pharmacology of paracetamol and NSAIDs

		Daily dose (mg)	Dose interval (h)	Elimination half-life (h)
Paracetamol		2000–4000	4	2
Salicyclates	Aspirin	1000–3600	4	0.25
	Diflunisal	500–1000	12–24	13
Acetic acids	Diclofenac	75–150	8	2
	Indomethacin	50–200	6–8	6
	Sulindac	300–400	12	15
	Etodolac	400–600	12–24	3
	Ketorolac	40–90	4–6	5
Propionic acids	Ibuprofen	1200–2400	6–8	2
	Fenbufen	900	12	10
	Flurbiprofen	150–300	12–24	4
	Ketoprofen	100–200	6–8	2
	Naproxen	500–1000	12	14
Fenamates	Mefenamic acid	750–1500	8	4
Oxicams	Piroxicam	20–40	12–24	60
	Tenoxicam	20	24	60
Phenylbutazone		300–400	6–8	60

mg/kg and the rectal dose is 20–25 mg/kg, with a daily maximum of 60 mg/kg. It is metabolized by the liver, conjugated with glucuronic and sulphuric acids, and excreted renally. Other minor metabolic pathways lead to problems if the drug is taken in overdose, when as little as 10 g can cause fatal hepatic or renal failure.

Salicylates are the oldest class of NSAIDs. Aspirin has an analgesic and antipyretic effect 10–30 minutes after a single dose; 3.6 g daily is needed to achieve anti-inflammatory actions. Side effects such as gastric irritation and tinnitus commonly occur at high doses and limit its usefulness as an NSAID. Enteric coated aspirin reduces occult gastro-intestinal bleeding, but has not been shown to affect symptoms such as dyspepsia and emesis. Renal excretion accounts for 10 per cent of each dose of aspirin. Excretion is increased when the urine is alkaline. Aspirin should be used with care in atopic patients as allergy is common. Aspirin should be avoided in children under 12 years because of the risk of potentially fatal Reye's syndrome. Benorylate is an ester of aspirin and paracetamol which is hydrolysed after ingestion to release both drugs. Diflunisal is a salicylate with a longer duration of action and a lower incidence of gut problems than aspirin.

Diclofenac is a phenylacetic acid that may be given orally, but has a lower bioavailability than most other NSAIDs (50 per cent). It is available as a slow release preparation. It can be given rectally. Parenteral diclofenac has been used in the treatment of acute and postoperative pain. It may produce pain at the site of injection. Diclofenac can be given to children over 12 months old (3 mg/kg/day in divided doses). Phenyl acetic acids are more likely to cause rashes than other NSAIDs.

Indoleacetic acids such as indomethacin, sulindac, and etodolac are well absorbed orally and rectally. Indomethacin is available as a slow release preparation which can be given at night to alleviate morning stiffness. It is extensively metabolized and may undergo enterohepatic recirculation. The use of indomethacin is limited by its side-effects. Sulindac may be preferable, as it has fewer side-effects and is less likely to lead to renal impairment. Etodolac may produce fewer gastrointestinal side-effects.

Ketorolac is a pyrroleacetic acid with good analgesic potency. It produces analgesia within 30 minutes of intramuscular injection which lasts for 4–6 hours. It can be administered intravenously and is used as a subcutaneous infusion in palliative care. The recommended dose was reduced after some patients experienced adverse effects. In acute pain or following surgery the initial parenteral dose is 10 mg followed by 10–30 mg every 4–6 hours. Parenteral treatment should only continue for 48 hours, with a maximum dose of 90 mg (60 mg in the elderly). It can be used orally in a dose of up to 40 mg for up to seven days.

Propionic acids, such as ibuprofen, fenbufen, flurbiprofen, ketoprofen, and naproxen have differing potencies and durations of action. Propionic acids are the best tolerated of all the NSAIDs. Ibuprofen has the fewest adverse effects of the gut, but is a weaker anti-inflammatory agent. Fenbufen is a prodrug. It can be given rectally to try to reduce adverse effects. Its long half life may lead to accumulation. Flurbiprofen is more potent, and penetrates synovial fluid better, but is more likely to cause gut problems.

Fenamates such as mefenamic acid have no particular advantages. They are more likely to cause nausea, vomiting, and diarrhoea. They are particularly contraindicated in inflammatory bowel disease.

Oxicams such as piroxicam and tenoxicam are long acting anti-inflammatory drugs that may be given once daily. They have a higher incidence of side-effects than other NSAIDs.

Pyrazoles such as phenylbutazone are potent anti-inflammatory drugs, but can produce serious blood dyscrasias. Their use is confined to specific situations such as inflammatory arthritides.

Adverse effects

The use of NSAIDs is often limited by the incidence of side-effects, which are particularly common in the elderly. There is a clear correlation between side-effects and long half life. Fatal complications are more common with the use of NSAIDs with a half life of 10 hours or greater. Patients should never be prescribed more than one NSAID at a time. The lower end of the dose range should be tried initially and titrated upwards. Acute soft tissue injury often responds to a short, orally administered course of a NSAID for 5–7 days. If the patient does not tolerate one class of NSAIDs, a drug from another group should be tried. In the treatment of chronic conditions such as back pain, and in the absence of side-effects, NSAIDs should be given at full dose for one to two weeks before they are being deemed ineffective.

The adverse effects of NSAIDs are largely due to their peripheral actions on prostaglandin synthesis. Reduced platelet function may increase bleeding, so aspirin and phenylbutazone are contraindicated in patients taking oral anticoagulants. Some NSAIDs such as ibuprofen or naproxen may be used if the prothrombin time is supervised carefully. NSAIDs adversely affect renal prostaglandin synthesis. They can cause chronic renal failure, acute interstitial nephritis, hyperkalaemic aldosteronism, and sodium and water retention. Risk factors for renal problems include old age, dehydration, shock, sepsis, heart failure, cirrhosis, and concommitant use of diuretics. NSAIDs should be used with caution in patients with a history of dyspepsia or peptic ulcers, as they may result in sudden severe gastrointestinal bleeding without preceding symptoms. Dyspepsia occurs in 10 per cent of those taking the newer NSAIDs; there is a higher incidence with aspirin and indomethacin. If NSAIDs are indicated it may be necessary to prescribe H_2-receptor blockers, proton pump inhibitors, or prostaglandin analogues (for example misoprostol) concurrently. Misoprostol may produce adverse effects such as nausea or diarrhoea and it is contraindicated in women of childbearing age. Gastrointestinal side-effects are related to the reduction of prostaglandin and prostacyclin synthesis and cannot be totally prevented by giving NSAIDs rectally or parenterally. Cyclo-oxygenase inhibition after NSAIDs results in a relative abundance of leukotrienes leading to hypersensitivity reactions such as urticaria, angio-oedema. Bronchospasm is common after aspirin and it occurs in 5–10 per cent of asthmatics. Most NSAIDs are relatively contraindicated in asthma. Non-specific side effects can occur after NSAIDs, such as headache, tinnitus, depression, dizziness, confusion, seizures, rashes, and psychological changes. Aspirin is contraindicated in children under 12 years old because of the risk of Reye's syndrome. NSAIDs should not be taken during pregnancy.

Pharmacology of antiemetics

Patients presenting for anaesthesia in the A & E department may be nauseated or vomiting because of illness, injury, gastric stasis, pain, or the administration of drugs such as opioids. The incidence of post-anaesthetic emesis depends on many factors including the drugs used, the type of surgery performed, and the propensity of the individuals to sickness. Prophylactic antiemetics are justified if the chance of emesis is high. Care must be taken that adverse effects from antiemetics are not produced in patients with only a low risk of emesis. Those at high risk should receive an antiemetic prophylactically. All patients using PCA devices should receive an antiemetic. The cause of nausea and vomiting should determine the class of antiemetic prescribed. If a prophylactic antiemetic fails to control the problem, then an antiemetic from a different group must be used. The site of action of antiemetics is often mixed and central cholinergic, dopaminergic, and serotoninergic transmission play an important role. Antiemetics should be given parenterally.

Physiology of emesis

Nausea is a subjective unpleasant sensation associated with the upper gastrointestinal tract. Vomiting involves expulsion of gastric contents from the mouth. It is often preceded by autonomic signs such as pallor, sweating and tachycardia. Vomiting comprises

- closure of the glottis to protect the lungs
- elevation of the soft palate to close entry to the nose
- contraction of the abdominal muscle to expel gastric contents.

The stomach does not contract during vomiting. Regurgitation is a passive process, which occurs when the consciousness level is depressed. It is more of a problem to the anaesthetist as it implies a lack of airway control with a risk of aspiration of gastric contents into the lungs. Nausea and vomiting can be relieved by drugs, but regurgitation is not affected by antiemetic medication (unless this has been used to try to reduce the volume of stomach contents).

Nausea and vomiting may be induced by various stimuli including pregnancy, acute pain, obesity, hypotension, hypoxaemia, raised intracranial pressure, psychological factors, labyrinthine disorders, metabolic disturbance, or gut irritation. Many different drugs can cause emesis, some via a gastric irritant effect, for example NSAIDs, and some via central mechanisms, for example opioids, digoxin, antibiotics, and neostigmine. The putative vomiting centre is in the medulla. It is activated by a variety of stimuli. These include nerve impulses from viscera, for example, pharyngeal stimulation, distension of the gut or biliary tract, and gastric mucosal irritation. A chemosensor, the chemoreceptor trigger zone (CTZ) is located in the medulla. The CTZ is exposed to drugs and chemicals in the blood and cerebrospinal fluid. Some drugs produce emesis via other mechanisms than the CTZ. Therefore antiemetics that act only at the CTZ are not effective for all types of emesis. The cerebral cortex affects the vomiting centre, therefore sights, smells, and psychological factors may cause vomiting. The vestibular system causes motion sickness. The cerebellum and CTZ are also involved.

Postoperative nausea and vomiting in children

The incidence of postoperative emesis in children may be up to 70 per cent. Emergency surgery, anxiety, and early mobilization and early fluid intake are predisposing factors. Newer anaesthetic agents such as sevoflurane may reduce the problem. The combination of local blocks and NSAIDs with anaesthesia reduces the need for opioids and decreases emesis. Prophylactic antiemetics should be used in high risk cases. Ondansetron may be useful in children and it has the advantage of having fewer side-effects than many of the other agents.

Classes of antiemetic drugs

Anticholinergic drugs

All drugs that antagonize the action of acetyl choline and can cross the blood–brain barrier have antiemetic properties (not glycopyrrolate). They are not active at the CTZ. They are useful in motion sickness and antagonize the emetic effects of opioids. They are more effective prophylactically than after emesis has occurred. Hyoscine, and some anti-histamines are most commonly used. Scopolamine (L-hyoscine) is well absorbed from the gut and can be used sublingually, subcutaneously, or as a transdermal patch. It has a short duration of action. It decreases lower oesophageal sphincter tone and reduces barrier pressure, therefore it may predispose to regurgitation. It produces autonomic side-effects such as dry mouth and pupillary dilation and has a sedative effect. It may cause confusion in elderly patients. Anticholinergic antiemetics are not ideal for the A & E setting.

Antihistamines

Antihistamines have antiemetic properties, examples include cinnarizine, cyclizine, dimenhydrinate, and promethazine. Sedation is a common side effect. Dry mouth, retention of urine, and drowsiness can occur. Anti-histamines that do not cross the blood–brain barrier, such as terfenadine, are not antiemetic.

Phenothiazines

These are useful in controlling emesis whether from drugs or other causes such as uraemia or radiotherapy. Many pheno-thiazines are also anticholinergic. Chloropromazine is an antiemetic, but its other effects such as sedation and hypotension limit its use. Methotrimeprazine is also anal-gesic. It is more sedative than chlorpromazine and is used in palliative care. Prochlorperazine is less sedative, because of the lack of anticholinergic action. A buccal preparation of Prochloperazine has been produced to improve bio-availability and prolong its action. It does not confer any advantages.

Buterophenones

Haloperidol is effective as an antiemetic, but it is long acting and takes several days to reach steady state concentrations. Droperidol has a shorter duration of action. It is commonly used with PCA machines to help emesis. It is not suitable for day cases.

Prokinetic antiemetics

Metoclopramide produces antiemesis via central antago-nism of dopamine. It has effects on the gut that are mediated cholinergically. It increases gastric emptying, relaxes the pylorus, and stimulates peristalsis. It increases lower oesophageal sphincter tone. It should not be given to patients with gastric outflow obstruction. It is well absorbed orally and has a short half life. Metoclopramide is often used to try to promote gastric emptying prior to surgery, but it cannot guarantee an empty stomach. Metoclopramide may cause extrapyramidal effects, especially in young people. Domperidone is less well absorbed after oral administration than metoclopramide, so a rectal preparation is commonly used. It is less likely to cause extrapyramidal side-effects than metoclopramide.

Anti-5-hydroxytryptamine (5-HT$_3$) drugs

Ondansetron and granisetron block 5-HT$_3$ centrally and in the vagal terminals in the gut. Ondansetron is rapidly absorbed after oral administration. It was originally used in prevention of post-radiation and cytotoxic-induced emesis.

It is now being used in postanaesthetic emesis and palliative care. The effect of a single dose persists for many hours. It has few side-effects.

Others
Cisapride is a prokinetic drug. It facilitates acetyl choline release at the myenteric plexus and has a gut-transit enhancing effect. It does not alter gut secretory function. It is used in oesophageal reflux, postprandial epigastric discomfort, and constipation. Benzodiazepines are used as antiemetics during chemotherapy. The amnesic action prevents anticipatory vomiting and they may modify central control of emesis. Steroids are used to treat nausea and vomiting in patients with cancer and during chemotherapy.

Treatment of acute dystonia

This may be manifest by trismus, torticollis, facial spasm, and oculogyric crisis and is more common in young women. It should not be mistaken for tetanus. Treatment with 1–2 mg of intravenous benztropine or 10 mg of intravenous procyclidine is effective, and may need repeating after 30 minutes.

Analgesia for specific situations
Children

Fear rather than pain may be a major cause for a child's distress, which may be potentiated by the accompanying adult, who may feel anxious, guilty, helpless, or angered by what has happened. The child's response will also be affected by previous experiences of hospital or what he or she has been told by family or friends. Many young children will be in the A & E department at a time when they would normally be asleep at home. Tiredness and hunger can reduce tolerance in both child and parent. Most children will settle with patient, sensitive handling and appropriate analgesia if required. There should be no major difference in the therapeutic approach to pain relief in children from that in adults. Analgesia should not be withheld because the child is unable to explain what the problem is. Children tolerate opioids well, and some can use Entonox effectively. Local anaesthetic techniques are acceptable to many children. Femoral nerve blocks are useful for fractured shafts of the femur. Some visually severe injuries, such as finger-tip injuries, may require little or no analgesia. Parenteral analgesia, such as intramuscular morphine, is often needed for the treatment of burns and scalds. Morphine has the advantage of having anxiolytic as well as analgesic properties. Children may go home after a single dose of morphine. Antiemetics may not be routinely needed with opioid analgesics in children. All drug doses must be carefully calculated, using the child's weight, and recorded. If a child does not settle he or she should be reassessed to exclude any other injury and determine the need for further analgesia. Sedation, for example with trimeprazine tartrate, should rarely be used. Premedication with oral midazolam 0.5–0.75 mg/kg mixed with paracetamol syrup (10 mg/kg) may be useful in distressed children prior to minor surgical procedures such as suturing under local anaesthetic. An uncontrollable child is likely to be in pain as well as being frightened. The use of intramuscular morphine is preferable, since it provides sedation and analgesia, and works more quickly than an oral drug.

Parents must be given simple, clear instructions about the use of analgesics at home. Many parents are reluctant or afraid to give analgesics to their child, particularly if she or he has had a head injury. Some parents regard paracetamol as a 'sleeping medication', possibly because the child is able to sleep once the pain has been relieved. Such misconceptions should be dispelled and appropriate advice should be given. Salicylate should never be given to children under twelve years old, because of its association with Reye's syndrome.

Acute abdominal pain

In the past it was common practice to withhold analgesia from patients with acute abdominal pain, in case it masked important abdominal signs. Some doctors still believe that it is preferable to leave the patient in pain, although patients and relatives think otherwise (Salter 1985). Analgesia is likely to be beneficial to patient and doctor. A pain-free patient is able to give a clearer history and examination is often facilitated, with tenderness and rigidity becoming more localized and masses more easily palpable (Attard *et al.* 1992). It is impossible to obtain good radiographs if the patient is restless with renal colic or pain from a perforated ulcer. Pain relief may be achieved with incremental intravenous doses of an opioid such as morphine. Non-steroidal anti-inflammatory drugs, given parenterally, give effective pain relief in renal and biliary colic (Hetherington and Philip 1986).

Multiple injuries

Entonox is the analgesic of choice for initial transport, assessment, and resuscitation following multiple injuries. The patient should then be given 100 per cent oxygen as soon as possible. Other analgesic techniques may be used once initial resuscitation is complete and the patient's condition is stable. These may include the use of splints, nerve blocks, or an intravenous opioid.

Head injuries

Control of the airway, breathing, and circulation take priority in any head injured patient. It is then essential to identify any life threatening intracranial injury, such as an extradural haematoma, which can be treated surgically. Analgesia may be given once the patient's condition is stable. The use of opioids is contentious. These may mask clinical signs that may indicate a deterioration in cerebral function. Pain is detrimental to the head injured patient, since it can cause an increase in intracranial pressure, which aggravates secondary brain injury. Pain, by making the patient restless and uncooperative, may mimic a deterioration in consciousness level. Pain may be the result of the head injury or of associated injuries, and thus will require different management in each of these cases. Headache has different origins, and its management is dependent on the severity of the injury.

Headache
Three types of headache may be associated with head injuries.

1. A moderate or severe generalized headache, which may be associated with vomiting or other neurological symptoms or signs, indicates the possibility of an intracranial haematoma. This pain may not be relieved by simple analgesics. A neurosurgical opinion should be sought. A computed tomography (CT) scan should be performed on patients suspected of having an intracranial haematoma.

2. Pain localized to the site of the injury and associated with bruising and swelling is relieved by simple oral analgesics suitable for mild pain, such as paracetamol. Pain usually settles within a few hours, although the area may still be tender to touch. Simple analgesics do not alter consciousness level or affect pupil size, nor are they strong enough to relieve the headache caused by raised intracranial pressure. A mild analgesic can therefore be given for the localized headache without fear of masking signs.

3. Pain due to an excessive intake of alcohol, which is common before a head injury, should respond to mild analgesics. Its persistence or an increase in severity should suggest the possibility of an intracranial haematoma.

Injuries associated with head injury

Patients with a head injury often have other injuries. Analgesics for mild or moderate pain may be given orally to the conscious patient. Severe pain may be relieved by a nerve block, intramuscular non-steroidal anti-inflammatory drugs, or small incremental intravenous doses of an opioid such as morphine. It should be possible, by careful use of the analgesic, to make the patient comfortable and still monitor consciousness level, making allowances for some change due to the analgesia. It should therefore still be possible to identify a deterioration in the patient's neurological state. If an intracranial lesion is suspected the patient should have a CT scan. The patient must have adequate analgesia for transfer to the scanning unit. The anaesthetist should be involved early in the management of these patients. It is often safer to anaesthetize and electively ventilate a head injured patient for an emergency CT scan. The anaesthetist should be involved immediately if a head injured patient begins to deteriorate.

Minor head injury (GCS 13 to 15)

These patients have a low risk of having an intracranial haematoma. The history, symptoms, and signs indicate the need for admission to hospital. A skull fracture is associated with an increased risk of intracranial haematoma. Headache is usually of the localized type that responds to mild analgesics. In young children, who are unable to indicate a headache, it is reasonable to assume that one may be present and to encourage parents to give paracetamol during the first twelve hours following injury.

Moderate head injury (GCS 9 to 12)

These patients will be admitted to hospital. Many will need a CT scan. They may show signs of pain from other injuries, and this should be treated using nerve blocks, intramuscular non-steroidal anti-inflammatory drugs, or small incremental intravenous doses of an opioid such as morphine. An anaesthetist should be involved early in their management, in case intubation and ventilation are required.

Severe head injury (GCS ⩽8)

These patients are unconscious and are generally assumed not to experience pain. They should be intubated and ventilated, and require an urgent CT scan. Patients under light general anaesthesia, although unconscious, may respond to stimuli such as pain or pharyngeal suction by, for example, lachrymating, coughing, or developing a tachycardia. It is possible that unconscious head injured patients also respond to similar stimuli, which may result in a dangerous increase in intracranial pressure. Elective intubation and ventilation must therefore be performed using an intravenous induction agent and a muscle relaxant. The patient should also be given an intravenous opioid if there are any injuries likely to cause pain. Complete sedation, analgesia, and muscle relaxation must be maintained.

Chest injuries

The initial priority is the maintenance of adequate oxygenation. Some chest injuries, such as a tension pneumothorax, are life threatening, and require immediate treatment which must take preference over attempts to provide analgesia.

Entonox may be used during transport and initial assessment of the patient. It should be avoided if a pneumothorax is suspected until a chest drain has been inserted. The patient should receive 100 per cent oxygen as soon as possible.

Chest injuries, particularly fractures of the ribs or sternum, are extremely painful. The pain restricts breathing, causing atelectasis, hypoxaemia, and hypercarbia, and may lead to infection. Oximetry and arterial blood gas measurement should be used to monitor the response to treatment. Incremental intravenous doses of an opioid may be given once the patient's condition is stable. Intercostal nerve blocks provide good analgesia for fractured ribs (see p. 370). Long term analgesia is best provided by a continuous local anaesthetic technique, maintained, for example, via intrapleural or thoracic epidural catheters. Patients should be admitted to the intensive care or high dependency unit if this technique is to be used. Adequate analgesia, oxygen therapy, and physiotherapy may be sufficient to manage a severe chest injury, but occasionally ventilation is required.

Minor chest injuries, involving the fracture of one or two ribs, can also be exceedingly painful and reduce ventilatory function. Initial pain may require parenteral analgesia or an intercostal nerve block. Patients receiving an intercostal nerve block may require admission to hospital so that this can be repeated. An oral analgesic for moderate pain should be prescribed to take at home. The pain from a fractured rib may persist for up to three months.

Abdominal and pelvic injury

Abdominal and pelvic trauma may be part of a complex multiple trauma problem, in which the first priority is always resuscitation and the treatment of life threatening conditions. Entonox may be used and incremental intravenous doses of an opioid may be administered once the patient's condition has stabilized.

Burns

Cold water is used in the emergency treatment of burns, to limit thermal injury, wash off chemical agents, and provide pain relief. Patients with extensive burns should never be immersed in cold water or have cold compresses applied, since this may cause hypothermia. Burns are less painful if the patient is treated in a warm, draught free room with the burn kept lightly covered to reduce evaporation. Partial thickness burns usually become pain free once an appropriate dressing is applied. Entonox may be used while the dressing is being done. Parenteral analgesia may be required for small children who cannot use Entonox. Although full thickness burns are superficially anaesthetic the overall effect of the burn and the burn edges and associated oedema can be extremely painful. Adequate analgesia must be provided. This is best given by incremental intravenous doses of an opioid such as morphine. The patient may also have thermal inhalation injuries. These can cause airway and ventilation problems, but should not preclude the use of analgesia. The anaesthetist should be called to discuss the need for intubation and ventilation of any patient with facial or neck burns, or of anyone who has inhaled smoke, steam, or chemicals.

Soft tissue injury

Physiotherapy can provide pain relief for some ligament and muscle sprains. It can also be effective in the management of whiplash injuries of the neck or torticollis. Oral non-steroidal anti-inflammatory analgesics may be beneficial in soft tissue injuries, the value of topical preparations is less certain. Transcutaneous electrical nerve stimulation is useful for soft tissue injuries. Benzydamine mouthwash is effective at relieving the discomfort of inflammatory mouth conditions, whether traumatic or infective. It may be used in babies who have feeding problems as a result of oral monilial infection.

Munchausen syndrome ('hospital-hoppers')

Patients with Munchausen syndrome appear to have an addiction to surgical or medical care. They repeatedly and convincingly feign a wide variety of illnesses in the hope of being admitted to hospital. They are typically young to middle-aged men whose employment allegedly requires nationwide travel. They may have many false names and addresses. They may 'collapse' in the street, or provide textbook descriptions of conditions such as renal colic, angina, or pulmonary embolism, which may normally require analgesia. Suspicion and experience are the key to identifying this problem. Senior nurses are often the first to recognize these patients. Some A & E departments have lists of 'hospital-hoppers', and it may be useful to discuss the problem with other departments, particularly in order to avoid misdiagnosing patients with typical histories who turn out to have genuine problems. Munchausen syndrome patients may also be genuinely ill at some stage. If the diagnosis is in doubt and parenteral analgesia seems necessary, intramuscular diclofenac may be given, since it has no sedative or addictive properties and the patient can be readily discharged after its use.

Drug addiction

Drug addicts will occasionally try to obtain their 'fix' from the A & E department. Since drugs are not available from this source addicts may pretend to have some painful condition, such as renal colic, which requires strong analgesia. Textbook descriptions are given, and physical signs may be present. Intramuscular diclofenac is useful in this situation, since it does not provide a 'fix', but does provide good analgesia for genuine renal colic. There will be situations where drug addicts genuinely need analgesia, and this must be chosen to fit the clinical situation. If an opioid is clinically indicated then it may be given, using an appropriate dose to provide adequate analgesia.

Prehospital care

Initial patient management should follow the 'ABC' of resuscitation within the limitations of the environment. Life-threatening conditions should be diagnosed and treated.

Prolonged and untreated pain may exacerbate shock. Severe pain causes an increase in circulating catecholamines, which produce vasoconstriction and reduce tissue perfusion. This counters the main aim of maintaining adequate tissue perfusion and oxygenation.

Entonox

Entonox is a commonly used analgesic for prehospital care. It takes about 30 seconds to start working and wears off within two minutes after discontinuing inhalation. It can be used in the majority of trauma cases. It should never be used to treat pain caused by the 'bends' (caisson disease), and must be used with caution in chest injuries where a pneumothorax is suspected. The presence of a chest drain makes its use less hazardous. Entonox may be used in head injured patients if other injuries are causing pain unless there is a compound skull fracture. It is not required in the unconscious patient. Entonox is effective in the treatment of myocardial pain, and hysterical overbreathing may be terminated by its use. Entonox may be used to control the pain from lower limb injuries, particularly during extrication or manipulation. Limbs may be relatively pain free while splinted by folded metal, but during release this splintage is lost, causing severe pain. It is essential to coordinate extrication with the rescuers. The patient should receive a three to four minute 'top up' of Entonox before the splinting metal is removed and the patient is freed. Patients should not suffer pain because the rescuers are too impatient or too lazy to use Entonox. The same 'saturation' technique may also be used before reducing fractures or dislocations at the scene of the accident in cases in which the circulation is threatened.

Parenteral analgesics

These may be required when Entonox is not suitable or ineffective on its own. They should always be given intravenously, in small incremental doses. Diamorphine, pethidine, or morphine may be used. Nalbuphine is sometimes used by paramedical staff as there is a ceiling to its ventilatory depressant effect. All can cause vomiting, ventilatory depression, and hypotension. An antiemetic should be given and naloxone must be available to reverse respiratory depression. Cyclimorph-10 (morphine 10 mg and cyclizine 50 mg/ml) is useful in prehospital care, being a premixed preparation of an analgesic and an antiemetic. Hypotension can be controlled by the administration of intravenous fluids. Opioid analgesics should not be given to patients with airway obstruction and are best avoided in the prehospital care of head injured patients. Ketorolac and diclofenac can be given intramuscularly in the head injured patient. Ketamine can be used in prehospital care if its benefits and limitations are remembered (see p. 90)

Regional analgesia

Regional techniques are useful for limb injuries. Nerve blocks allow pain free movement of limbs and facilitate the reduction of fractures or the application of splints. The techniques should be practised in a controlled hospital environment before they are used in prehospital care, where optimal positioning may be impossible. The doctor should choose the local anaesthetic with which she or he is most familiar for each particular block. It is essential to know the maximum safe doses for all ages, and how to identify and treat toxic reactions. Regional blocks are discussed in detail in the section on local anaesthesia.

Sedation

Occasionally, anxious or hysterical patients may require sedation. However, hypoxaemia, hypovolaemia, head injury, or severe pain can mimic these states and should be excluded before any sedation is given. A small dose of Diazemuls (2– 10 mg) given slowly intravenously, may be used; but this is long acting and can cause ventilatory depression. Midazolam (1–5 mg) intravenously may be more useful, having a shorter duration of action. Benzodiazepines may cause hypotension in the elderly and must be given in small doses. Small doses of haloperodol may be as effective.

Chronic pain

Acute pain must be distinguished from chronic pain. The former acts to warn of and protect from impending tissue damage, and the latter seems to serve no biological function. Patients usually present to the A & E department with acute pain conditions which are self-limiting, and may result in acute anxiety. Patients with chronic pain are more likely to be depressed and may come to the A & E department because of an acute exacerbation of pain or because of a failure to cope. It must be remembered that they may also present with an entirely new pain problem.

Chronic pain is defined as a 'pain that persists beyond the usual course of an acute disease or beyond the reasonable time for an injury to heal'. Chronic pain may result from persistent pathological problems in somatic structures or viscera, or from prolonged dysfunction of peripheral or central nerves. It may occur in benign or malignant diseases. It may be associated with psychological, environmental, and social factors. As well as being a health problem, chronic pain places a major socio-economic burden on industrialized countries, where it is estimated that chronic pain syndromes may afflict 30 per cent of the population.

Patients with chronic pain should be assessed in the same systematic way as those with acute pain. It is easy to be dismissive of patients with a 'chronic pain' label. It is important to ensure that the problem that they have attended the A & E department with does not require urgent treatment. If a history and examination suggest that the pain is not new, it is important to decide whether the condition of the patient warrants admission to hospital.

Patients with cancer pain who present to the A & E department may require admission to hospital. It is not appropriate to give these patients one dose of parenteral opioid and send them home. The fact that they have attended hospital suggests that they and their family are not coping. Referral to specific agencies, such as Macmillan nurses, hospital support teams, hospices, and home care teams may be needed. This should be coordinated with the help of the general practitioner, once the immediate problem of severe pain has been sorted out.

Patients with 'benign' chronic pain conditions (Table 11.4) may occasionally need admission to hospital; for example, very elderly patients may not be able to manage at home, and those who are socially isolated may be at risk of suicide. If the problem does not warrant admission then the patient should be given simple pain relieving measures and referred to the doctor who normally treats their pain problem. Opioid analgesics are sometimes used for 'benign' chronic pain, but the decision to commence long term use should be made by the pain specialist or the general practi-

Table 11.4 c Common chronic pain conditions

- Low back pain
- Facial pain (migraine, trigeminal neuralgia, atypical facial pain)
- Postherpetic neuralgia
- Post-traumatic pain (scar pain, stump pain)
- Phantom limb pain
- Sympathetically mediated pain (reflex sympathetic dystrophy, causalgia)
- Centrally mediated pain (pain following a stroke)
- Cancer pain

tioner, and not by a doctor who does not know the patient and may never see him or her again. If the patient is attending a pain management clinic it is important that the appropriate consultant and the general practitioner are informed of the patient's attendance at the A & E department.

Further reading

Attard A. R., Corlett, M. J., Kichen, N. J., Leslie, A. B., and Fraser I. A.(1992). Safety of early pain relief for acute abdominal pain. *British Medical Journal*, **305**, 554–6.

Beyer, J. E. and Wells, N. (1989). The assessment of pain in children. *Paediatric Clinics of North America*, **36**, 837–54.

Hetherington, J. W. and Philip, N. H. (1986). Diclofenac sodium versus pethidine in acute renal colic. *British Medical Journal*, **292**, 237–8.

Lloyd-Thomas, A. R. (1990). Pain management in paediatric patients. *British Journal of Anaesthesia*, **64**, 85–104.

Reichl, M. and Bodiwalla, C. G. (1987). The use of analgesia in severe pain in the A & E department. *Archives of Emergency Medicine*, **4**, 25–31.

Salter, R. H. (1985). Diagnosis before treatment? *Lancet*, **i**, 863–4.

Selbst, S. M. (1989). Managing pain in the paediatric emergency department. *Paediatric Emergency Care*, **5**, 56–63.

Strom, B. L., Berlin, J. A., and Kinman, J. L. (1986). Parenteral ketorolac and the risk of gastrointestinal and operative site bleeding. *Journal of the American Medical Association*, **275**, 376–82.

White, P. F. (1988). Pain management after day case surgery. *Current opinion in Anaesthesia*, **1**, 70–5.

Wilson, J. E. and Pendleton, J. M. (1989). Oligoanalgesia in the emergency department. *American Journal of Emergency Medicine*, **7**, 620–3.

Yates, D. W. (1984). Mild analgesics and the accident and emergency department—cost and safety more important than potency? *Archives of Emergency Medicine*, **1** 197–203.

Part 4
Local anaesthesia

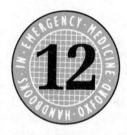

CHAPTER 12

Local anaesthesia: principles and practice in the A & E department

---

Key points in local anaesthesia: principles and practice in the A & E department

- Obtain a brief medical history and record medication and allergies, since these may affect the choice of local anaesthetic drug or technique

- Double-check the drug labels before drawing up the solution, particularly if adrenaline is contraindicated

- Before injecting any local anaesthetic check the maximum dose which may be used and be particularly careful in children

- Local anaesthetic should always be injected slowly

- Stop injecting immediately if the injection becomes painful or the patient develops symptoms of toxicity, such as tinnitus or tingling around the mouth

- Record legibly precise details of the anaesthetic technique, including the type and amount of local anaesthetic used

- Certain more complex techniques such as brachial plexus block require practice and should probably be restricted to experienced practitioners.

Introduction

Local anaesthetic techniques form an essential part of practice in A & E medicine. The techniques should provide good pain control, with minimal discomfort or danger to the patient. They are used most commonly to aid wound cleansing and closure. They are invaluable in the management of pain, but are often under used in this situation. Local anaesthesia is cheap, simple, and relatively safe, and is often the technique of choice for patients in poor general health. It may be used in unfasted patients, although fasting is necessary for intravenous regional anaesthesia and blocks involving large doses of local anaesthetic. Many techniques can be performed by well-trained A & E doctors without the help of an anaesthetist.

Local anaesthesia has its limitations. It is not as reliable as general anaesthesia, particularly in obese patients. Operations may be restricted by the limit on the dose of local anaesthetic which can be used, and some patients will not tolerate being awake during an operation.

Indications and contraindications

Indications

- Any situation where local anaesthesia will provide safe, adequate operating conditions or satisfactory analgesia
- Patients with a poor medical history, such as pulmonary disease
- Possible problems with maintaining an airway, although high doses of local anaesthetic should also be avoided, because of the risk of toxicity causing airway problems
- Previous adverse reactions to general anaesthesia

Contraindications

- Refusal or poor cooperation from the patient.
- Allergy to local anaesthetic. It may be possible to choose a safe drug from a different group of local anaesthetics.

Multi-dose vials should not be used if there is a history of allergy to a local anaesthetic, in case the allergy is caused by the preservative used in these preparations.

- Infection at the site of injection. Injection of local anaesthetic through or into infected tissue is often painful, and risks spreading infection. The high tissue acidity may reduce the local anaesthetic effect. The increased vascularity of infected tissue may speed up absorption of local anaesthetic, causing a toxic reaction. However, it is possible to anaesthetize small abscesses by circumferential local infiltration a distance away from the abscess without any adverse reaction or clinical sign of spread of infection.

- Anticoagulant therapy or bleeding diathesis (prothrombin time greater than 1.5 times control or platelets less than $50 \times 10^9/l$). The main risk lies in accidental arterial puncture.

Special caution

- Extremes of age
- Debilitated patients
- Low cardiac output
- Impaired cardiac conduction
- Hepatic impairment
- Epilepsy
- Myasthenia gravis

In all the above situations there may be an increased risk of developing a toxic reaction. It is essential to choose the type of block and local anaesthetic carefully, and to monitor the heart rate, blood pressure, and respiratory rate. The dose of local anaesthetic should generally be reduced.

- Neurological disease, where an exacerbation may be blamed on the local anaesthetic. This is of relevance particularly to the use of nerve blocks involving a previously affected area. The problem is more medico-legal than practical.

Local anaesthesia and children

The basic principles of local anaesthetic techniques in children are the same as for adults. It is vital that every A & E doctor masters these, so that children are not deprived of the benefits of local anaesthesia. Femoral nerve blocks are useful in providing analgesia for a fractured shaft of the femur in children of any age (see p. 346). The block may be performed before the diagnosis is confirmed by radiography and will allow painless immobilization of the leg in a splint. An ulnar nerve block can provide anaesthesia for the reduction of a displaced fracture of the little finger. Infiltration anaesthesia may be used for suturing wounds, but its use can be kept to a minimum with the use of adhesive skin closure, as with Steristrips or skin glue. In some cases local anaesthesia will be required to provide adequate wound toilet.

Some doctors are apprehensive about using local anaesthesia on children. This is often due to inexperience in dealing with young children. Local anaesthetic techniques should only be performed on children by experienced doctors, preferably with the assistance of an experienced nurse. The dose of the drug should be calculated carefully (Tables 12.1, 12.2). Smaller needles than those used for adults are required. It is also helpful to use the smallest

Table 12.1 • Maximum safe doses of solutions of local anaesthetics without vasoconstrictor

Drug	Dose (mg/kg)*
Esters	
Cocaine	2–3
Procaine	7
Amethocaine	1.0–1.5
Amides	
Bupivacaine	2
Lignocaine	4
Prilocaine	6
Mepivacaine	4
Ropivacaine	2

* These doses are only approximate and refer to a single dose given into a non-vascular area. The doses of some anaesthetics may sometimes be increased by the use of adrenaline.

Table 12.2 • Dosage chart of lignocaine and bupivacaine

Patient's weight (kg)	1% lignocaine plain, 4 mg/kg (ml)	1% lignocaine with adrenaline, 7 mg/kg (ml)	0.5% bupivacaine plain,* 2 mg/kg (ml)
10	4	7	4
20	8	14	8
30	12	21	12
40	16	28	16
50	20	35	20
60	24	42	24
70	28	49	28
80	32	56	32
90	36	63	36
100	40	70	40

* The addition of adrenaline does not increase the maximum permissible dose of bupivacaine.

possible syringe for the local anaesthetic, since it will be less intimidating to the child and will reduce the chance of giving an overdose. All the equipment should be prepared and then put out of view before the child enters the room. In this way the environment will be less frightening for the child and mistakes in drawing up the local anaesthetic are less likely to occur. It is vital to win the confidence and cooperation of the child and any accompanying adult. The procedure should be explained simply and honestly. It is far better to say that something may feel uncomfortable than to mislead the child. Appropriate paediatric resuscitation equipment should be available when local anaesthetics are given to children. The doctor should be familiar with the equipment and with the dose of emergency drugs which may be required. If satisfactory conditions cannot be obtained and an anaesthetic is required then a general anaesthetic would usually be the method of choice.

General principles of local anaesthetic techniques

A nerve fibre may be blocked by local anaesthetic at any level, from the spinal cord within the dura to the sensory receptor at the periphery. Local anaesthetic must diffuse into the cell membrane to produce its effect. The speed with which this occurs will depend on the degree of myelination, the size of the nerve, and the relative position of the fibre within the nerve. Thus a nerve fibre may be rapidly blocked by a spinal anaesthetic, but the same fibre will take much longer to be anaesthetized once it is part of a major nerve such as the femoral nerve. Infiltration of local anaesthetic peripherally will again produce a rapid effect on the nerve fibre by acting on its sensory nerve endings.

A block at spinal cord level will affect many segments and produce a large area of anaesthesia with a dermatomal pattern. As the block is placed more peripherally, smaller areas are involved, which represent the area of supply of the peripheral nerve. After local infiltration only those nerve endings directly in contact with the local anaesthetic will be anaesthetized, thus the area of anaesthesia will depend upon the area of infiltration.

Local infiltration

This is the most commonly used technique in the A & E department. The local anaesthetic is injected subcutaneously at the site of the sensory nerve endings. Only a small area is anaesthetized. Onset is within about 2 minutes, but the local anaesthetic is quickly removed by absorption into the circulation. Anaesthesia may therefore only last for 30 minutes, but can be prolonged if a vasoconstrictor is used. The technique uses relatively large volumes of local anaesthetic, for example, 5.0 ml of local anaesthetic may be required to anaesthetize a small knee laceration before suturing, whereas the same volume could produce an ulnar nerve block sufficient to treat a compound fracture of the little finger. The risk of toxicity can be reduced by using a low concentration of local anaesthetic, such as 0.5 per cent lignocaine and by using local anaesthetic with adrenaline where appropriate. Before injecting any local anaesthetic always check the maximum dose which may be used, and be particularly careful with children.

Field block

This uses an infiltration technique. A wall of local anaesthetic is injected subcutaneously around the operative field.

It relies on the fact that branches of the sensory nerves usually run parallel to the skin surface in the subcutaneous tissue. The technique may be used for the incision and drainage of a small abscess, or for cleaning small areas of gravel burn. It may also be more appropriate for dealing with ragged, dirty wounds, where injection well away from the wound edge is advantageous. Always check the maximum safe dose before starting a field block.

Nerve blocks

These are also commonly used in the A & E department, both for operative procedures (such as suturing the palm under a median nerve block) and for providing analgesia (as with a femoral nerve block for a fractured shaft of the femur).

Major nerve block (for example, of the femoral nerve)
The block of a major nerve will produce a large area of anaesthesia compared with the small area affected by an infiltration technique. Diffusion of local anaesthetic to all fibres will be slow, because of the size of the nerve, and anaesthesia may take up to 40 minutes to be established. Choosing the correct dose and volume of local anaesthetic is therefore very important. The local anaesthetic is removed slowly from the nerve, and thus the block may last for several hours. Large doses of local anaesthetic may be needed, and care must be taken to check the maximum safe dose.

Minor nerve block (for example, of ulnar or digital nerves)
This may be used for minor operative techniques or for providing analgesia, for example for a crushed finger. The area anaesthetized will not be as great as with the major nerve block. The smaller size of nerve will mean that anaesthetic onset will be more rapid – within 5 to 10 minutes – but will not last as long – perhaps up to 1 hour. Smaller doses of local anaesthetic are required.

Plexus block (for example brachial plexus)
Major nerves are blocked simultaneously where they all come together within an accessible anatomical site. The

comments regarding major nerve blocks are also applicable to plexus blocks.

Intravenous regional anaesthesia (IVRA: 'Bier's block')

This technique is often used instead of general anaesthesia for reducing fractures at the wrist. Anaesthesia is produced by injecting local anaesthetic into the venous system in the hand after first exsanguinating the limb and occluding arterial and venous flow with a tourniquet around the upper arm. The local anaesthetic diffuses out of the veins and through the tissue to the nerve endings. Anaesthetic action is first noted on the unmyelinated autonomic nerves, producing a mottling of the skin. Analgesia is established within 5 minutes. Once the tourniquet is released anaesthesia remains for a variable length of time as the local anaesthetic is absorbed back into the circulation. Local anaesthetic doses near the maximum safe limit are required. This technique should only be performed by those thoroughly trained in its use. For further discussion of IVRA see p. 315, 348.

Topical anaesthesia

Local anaesthetic is applied directly to the mucous membrane or skin, through which it diffuses to reach the sensory nerve endings. Onset of anaesthesia may therefore be slow. The drug is rapidly removed, and thus duration of action will be short. Topical anaesthetic preparations contain a high concentration of local anaesthetic, such as 4 per cent lignocaine. It is very easy to give a toxic dose. Topical anaesthesia is commonly used in the A & E department for removal of foreign bodies from the eye or for urethral catheterization. Its use for cleaning gravel burns can cause problems, as anaesthesia is rarely adequate to allow thorough wound toilet. It is much better to use a field block or a regional block for wound toilet. On occasions a general anaesthetic may be required.

Spinal and epidural anaesthesia

These techniques are unsuitable for A & E use, but are very important forms of regional anaesthesia in other clinical settings.

General procedure for local anaesthetic techniques

It is important to check that all the necessary equipment, including that for resuscitation, is available before starting the procedure. It is essential to be aware of the possible complications and their management. A plan of action should the block fail is also useful. Always obtain a brief medical history and record medication and allergies, as these may affect the choice of local anaesthetic or block.

Decide on the type of block to be used, and check the anatomical landmarks. Select the appropriate local anaesthetic, and decide whether adrenaline should be used. Calculate the maximum dose which may be given (Tables 12.1, 12.2, p. 274), and then the amount to be used initially. Ensure this does not exceed the maximum safe volume. Always double-check the drug labels before drawing up the solution, particularly if adrenaline is contraindicated. It is probably best to draw up initially only the expected dose required. This reduces the risk of giving an overdose. The size of syringe will depend on the volume of drug needed, the type of block, and personal preference for what is most easy to handle. Large syringes may be frightening to children and should be avoided in paediatric use.

It is essential to have the patient's consent and cooperation. Explain the procedure simply. The patient should understand that the initial injection may produce a stinging or burning sensation. Once the local anaesthetic is working there should be no pain, although sensations such as pressure may be felt. Describe the anticipated area of sensory loss. Patients often expect a very large area to be anaesthetized, and are worried if they have normal sensation near the operation site. Their confidence is strengthened by a correct prediction.

Intravenous access should be established before undertaking intravenous regional anaesthesia. It is also necessary if the maximum local anaesthetic dose may be used, if adjuvant intravenous medication is needed, or if the patient is at risk of having a toxic reaction (see p. 292).

Preparation and injection should follow normal aseptic

practice. Avoid recapping the needle because of the risk of a needle-stick injury. Always note the time of injection. An initial skin wheal may be raised with a 25-gauge needle before changing to a larger 22-gauge needle for the main injection. About 2 minutes may be needed for the initial infiltration to take effect. A larger gauge needle enables an easier injection and reduces the risk of needle breakage sometimes seen with finer needles. A slow injection will minimize discomfort and reduce the risk of a toxic reaction. Aspiration each time the needle is moved is essential to avoid intravascular injection. Small veins may collapse under negative pressure, so never assume that an injection is extravascular because there is no blood on aspiration. Resistance to injection may be due to nerve, tendon sheath, or periosteum, and the needle should be repositioned. Paraesthesiae in the peripheral distribution of the nerve may occur if the needle touches the nerve. Injection should not commence until the needle has been withdrawn slightly, since direct injection into the nerve may cause permanent nerve damage. Eliciting paraesthesiae can be a helpful way of identifying a nerve; but it should not be used routinely, because it is unpleasant for the patient, and may cause nerve damage.

Estimate when the block should be working, and only then test sensation. Testing too soon will reduce the patient's confidence. Needles are commonly used to test for analgesia, but the patient should always be distracted while this is done. The sight of a needle being pressed into the skin may be enough for a patient, particularly a child, to complain of pain despite there being an adequate block. It is often helpful to let the patient check the block for himself or herself by simple fingertip pressure. Never ask the patient if he or she feels pain when the operation is started, as it will be perfectly clear if the block is not working. It may be more pleasant for the patient if the adequacy of a block is assessed by testing cold sensation with ice. Decide whether the patient will need postoperative analgesia, and if so give the first dose before the block has worn off. Always record legibly the time, the site of injection, and the dose of anaesthetic used.

This book contains descriptions of local anaesthetic techniques which may be used in an A & E department. The doses quoted apply to the average '70 kg man', and corrections for age or associated medical conditions should be made where appropriate. The needle sizes have been chosen with regard to those most commonly available in an A & E department. It may be useful to have a separate limited supply of specialized needles. Many of the blocks may be used on children, and in some cases specific reference has been made to this. For children's doses see p. 275. Some techniques will be used every day, while others will only be needed in an emergency. This section does not include every block which may be used in the A & E department – for example, dental blocks have not been described. These may be of value, but are rarely required, and should only be performed after training.

The majority of the techniques listed below may be performed by a well trained A & E senior house officer, but a few of the techniques should be left to doctors with anaesthetic training. Anyone performing a local anaesthetic technique should be aware of the general principles (see p. 279) and have some basic knowledge of complications and their management (see p. 290). All should be proficient in basic life support. Resuscitation equipment should be available. The following are suggested as guidelines for managing local anaesthetic techniques.

Techniques requiring anaesthetic expertise

- Intravenous regional anaesthesia (IVRA)
- Brachial plexus blocks
- 3 in 1 block
- Sciatic nerve block
- Stellate ganglion block
- Topical anaesthesia of the larynx and trachea

Techniques requiring patient observation or admission after the block

- IVRA
- Femoral nerve block
- Intercostal nerve block
- Brachial plexus blocks (depending on site)
- 3 in 1 block
- Sciatic nerve block
- Stellate ganglion block
- Topical anaesthesia of the larynx and trachea

Techniques requiring a fasted patient

- IVRA
- Brachial plexus blocks
- 3 in 1 block
- Sciatic nerve block
- Stellate ganglion block
- Topical anaesthesia of the larynx and trachea

Techniques unsuitable for children

- IVRA (younger than eight years old)
- Infiltration of fracture haematoma
- Interscalene and subclavian perivascular brachial plexus block
- Stellate ganglion block
- Topical anaesthesia of larynx and trachea

Peripheral nerve stimulators and needles for nerve blocks

A peripheral nerve stimulator (PNS) can be used to locate nerves during nerve blocks by producing electrical stimulation via a needle. The larger the nerve fibre, the more readily it will be stimulated from any given distance. Mixed peripheral nerves can be located by producing twitch rather than parathesia. The use of a motor response rather than sensory perception reduces ambiguity. The stimulus required varies with the distance of the stimulating needle from the nerve. As the needle approaches the nerve the current needed to produce a response falls in an inverse square manner. Stimulation of a nerve from a distance of 2 cm requires a current of about 50 mA. Once the needle is on the nerve 0.5–1.0 mA is sufficient to evoke a twitch. Therefore by varying the current used for stimulation the distance of the needle from the nerve can be inferred.

Characteristics of PNS machines

Many small battery operated nerve stimulators are available, and the ideal machine should have the following features:

- A constant current output which does not vary with changes in the resistance of the external circuit (tissues, needles, and connectors).
- A clear display of the current delivered on a digital meter which reads as low as 0.5 mA.
- An easily movable output control with a linear scale.
- Leads with clearly marked polarity. The negative should be attached to the stimulating needle, and the positive to a ground electrode.
- A short pulse width, for example 50–200 μs, to provide better discrimination of the distance of the needle from the nerve.
- An optimum pulse frequency of 0.5–2.0 Hz.
- A battery indicator.
- High quality, low resistance alligator clips to allow use with a variety of needles.

Needles for nerve blocks

Ordinary injection needles can be used for skin infiltration. When performing blocks involving larger nerves, pencil point needles or needles with a 45° bevel are less traumatic. These are less likely to penetrate nerves than cutting needles. However, there is some evidence that if these needles do pierce nerves, they may produce more damage than conventional needles. Early reports of the use of PNS involved insulated needles. Ordinary metal needles can be used if the electrical differences between these and insulated needles are understood. Insulated needles are designed to concentrate the current density around the needle point. Once an insulated needle is more than 1 cm deep, the depth of insertion has no further effect on the current. Uninsulated metal needles have the maximum current density just proximal to the tip and extending up the needle's shaft. Unsheathed needles have a resistance and an electrical field pattern which varies with the depth of insertion. These factors may lead to inaccurate localization of nerves because of stimulation from the uninsulated needle shaft when the tip is beyond the nerve. Insulated needles are therefore more accurate and require less current than ordinary needles but they are more expensive, and do alter the 'feel' of injection. Ordinary metal needles are readily available and cheaper, but require more current and may be less accurate.

Technique for the use of PNS

1. Position the patient for the nerve block and identify the usual anatomical landmarks.
2. Insert the needle through an anaesthetized skin wheal and advance it for a short distance.
3. Connect the negative lead of the stimulator to the needle and the positive lead to a ground electrode (an ECG electrode is suitable).
4. Turn on the stimulator with a current of 2–5 mA, which may produce a localized muscle twitch (especially with uninsulated needles).
5. Advance the needle towards the desired nerve and look for motor movement in appropriate groups of muscles (for example, knee extension during femoral nerve stimulation).

6. Once muscle movement occurs the needle is 1–2 cm from the nerve. Advance the needle further towards the nerve and simultaneously reduce the current strength. Position the needle so that a twitch occurs with a current of 0.5–1.0 mA. The needle is now within a few millimetres of the nerve.

7. Give a test injection of 2 ml of local anaesthetic down the needle. If the needle is accurately placed the twitch will reduce or disappear within 10 seconds (probably because of physical displacement of the nerve). If the twitch does not alter after the test dose, reposition the needle using the PNS and repeat the test dose.

8. Once the abolition of the twitch by a test dose has confirmed accurate needle placement, the total volume of local anaesthetic should be injected.

PNS is useful as an aid to performing nerve blocks and when teaching, but should be used as an adjunct to good clinical practice and a sound knowledge of anatomy.

Further reading

Arthur, D. S. and McNicol, L. R. (1986). Local anaesthetic techniques in paediatric surgery. *British Journal of Anaesthesia*, **58**, 760–78.

Pither, C. E., Raj, P. P., and Ford, D. (1985). The use of peripheral nerve stimulators for regional anaesthesia. *Regional Anesthesia*, **10**, 49–58.

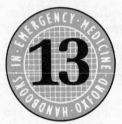

CHAPTER 13

Pharmacology of local anaesthetics

Key points in pharmacology of local anaesthetics

- Bupivacaine provides more prolonged anaesthesia and analgesia than lignocaine.

- Transdermal local anaesthetics such as EMLA cream or amethocaine gel can be useful, especially in paediatric anaesthesia.

- Adrenaline may be used with some local anaesthetics to reduce systemic absorption and bleeding and prolong anaesthesia. Adrenaline must never be used near end-arteries, such as fingers, toes, ear, nose, and penis.

All local anaesthetics have a similar chemical structure, a lipophilic aromatic ring linked to a hydrophilic amino moiety by a carbon chain. They exist as D and L isomers which may have stereospecificity in absorption and distribution, with implications for efficacy and safety. An example is ropivacaine which is presented as the single L isomer. It is similar to bupivacaine but produces less motor block and is less toxic. Local anaesthetics can be classified by the type of linkage – esters, for example cocaine, procaine, and amethocaine; and amides, for example lignocaine, bupivacaine, and prilocaine. Local anaesthetics can be used topically, (conjunctiva, mucous membranes) transdermally, by infiltration, for intravenous regional anaesthesia, to block nerves or nerve plexuses, and spinally.

Local anaesthetic drugs prevent nerve conduction by blocking sodium channels in axonal membranes. The neuronal block achieved also depends upon the structure of the nerves. Individual fibres vary in their degree of myelinization, speed of conduction, and susceptibility to blockade. The block produced by application of a local anaesthetic is also influenced by the relative position of the fibres within a nerve bundle, the outer most fibres being blocked first. Sympathetic nerves are blocked more easily than pain, temperature, and touch fibres, which are more susceptible than pressure, proprioception, and motor nerve fibres. It is possible to produce analgesia without motor block. If analgesia is present, sympathetic block will usually occur.

Potency, speed of onset, and duration of action

Effects of local anaesthetics depend upon their physio-chemical properties (Table 13.1). Local anaesthetics equilibrate rapidly across membranes because they are lipid soluble. They have large volumes of distribution. At a steady rate only a small proportion of the drug is confined to plasma. They are bound to plasma proteins, mainly α_1 acid glycoprotein. In a situation where local anaesthetics are injected rapidly, binding is not of major importance in relation to toxicity.

Potency increases with increased lipid solubility, for

Table 13.1 • Physico-chemical properties of local anaesthetics

	Lipid solubility	Relative potency	Protein binding	Duration of action	pK_a	Onset * (min)
Esters						
Procaine	Low	1	6%	Short	8.9	18
Amethocaine	High	8	76%	Long	8.5	15
Amides						
Bupivacaine	High	8	95%	Long	8.1	10
Lignocaine	Medium	2	64%	Medium	7.9	5
Prilocaine	Medium	2	55%	Medium	7.9	5
Mepivacaine	Low	2	77%	Medium	7.6	3
Ropivacane	High	8	94%	Long	8.1	10

* After infiltration larger nerve trunks take longer to anaesthetize.

example, bupivacaine is more potent than lignocaine (Table 13.1). The speed of onset is related to the degree of ionization at physiological pH, the diffusibility across membranes, and the concentration gradient developed between the site of injection and the site of action. Local anaesthetics are weak bases which are poorly soluble in water, and are presented for injection as hydrochloride salts. The free base diffuses to the site of action. The cation is the active agent. The degree of ionization is dependent on the pK_a of the drug. For example at pH 7.4 bupivacaine (pK_a 8.1) is very ionized and less diffusible, with a slower onset, than lignocaine (pK_a 7.9). As the pH falls, local anaesthetics become more ionized and less diffusible. They cannot easily get to the site of action in acid conditions, such as infection. The dose (volume $\times$ concentration) of local anaesthetic administered influences the onset, depth and duration of the block. The individual volume and concentration are unimportant, for example 60 mg of prilocaine gives the same result whether given as 3 ml of a 2 per cent solution or 6 ml of 1 per cent. However, an increase in the volume administered may sometimes affect the block by extending the spread of local anaesthetic. The site of injection alters the speed of onset and duration of the block; for example subcutaneous infiltration anaesthesia begins rapidly and is short lived, but plexus anaesthesia often starts slowly and may last for many hours.

The duration of action increases with increased protein binding. It is also influenced by the intrinsic vasoactive effect of the drug. For example, lignocaine causes more vasodilatation than prilocaine and is therefore shorter acting. The duration of action of local anaesthetics depends upon the rate of removal from the site of action by bulk flow during injection and diffusion, which is influenced by local blood flow. Local anaesthetics are more readily absorbed from inflamed areas. Injection into vascular sites increases the risk of a toxic reaction. The duration of effect of local anaesthetics limits their use for postoperative pain relief. The development of liposomal local anaesthetics may allow a slow release of drug with prolonged effects and reduced toxicity.

Metabolism

Ester local anaesthetics are rapidly removed by plasma cholinesterases and liver metabolism. Amide local anaesthetics are cleared by the liver. Total clearance is dependent on hepatic blood flow, binding, and enzyme function. Most amide local anaesthetics are potentially more toxic than esters. Prilocaine is metabolized in the liver, kidney, and lungs to o-toluidine and nitrosotoluidine which oxidize haemoglobin to methaemoglobin. Large doses of prilocaine may lead to methaemoglobinaemia. Local anaesthetics with large chemical groups, for example bupivacaine, resist hydrolysis, and are therefore longer acting. Renal excretion of unchanged local anaesthetics is minimal.

Transdermal local anaesthetics

The use of transdermal local anaesthesia has changed paediatric anaesthesia. There is now no reason for venepuncture to be painful. This technique is also useful in adults with needle phobia and for taking small skin grafts. A eutectic mixture of 2.5 per cent lignocaine and 2.5 per cent prilocaine bases produces a cream (EMLA) which can be used on the skin. The high concentration of uncharged base diffuses through the skin to produce analgesia. The cream must be applied thickly under an occlusive dressing and left for 60 minutes. The prolonged period of application is a disadvantage in the A & E setting, but with good anticipation of the need for injection this can be managed. Another problem is that the dressing leads to some skin oedema which may make the veins more difficult to see. The dressing and cream should be removed about 10 minutes before injection to reduce this problem. Transdermal 4 per cent amethocaine gel works more rapidly, in about 30 minutes, and may enable veins to be seen more easily. This could have advantages in the emergency setting.

Additives

Local anaesthetics can produce serious cardiovascular and central nervous toxicity. There are various ways to reduce the risks. The most important are to keep to the safe dose, use slow injection, maintain verbal contact with the patient, and use adequate monitoring. Adrenaline can be added to local anaesthetics to try to increase the speed of onset and duration of action and to reduce bleeding. Concentrations of more than 5 μg/ml (1:200000) are not necessary and can lead to toxicity (the maximum safe dose of adrenaline for a healthy adult is 500 μg). A high concentration of adrenaline (1:80000) is commonly used in dental anaesthesia. The use of adrenaline increases the duration of action of short and intermediate acting local anaesthetics by inducing local vasoconstriction; but differences are less apparent with long acting agents. Adrenaline decreases plasma levels and toxicity when added to lignocaine or mepivacaine; but the effect on bupivacaine absorption is less certain. Adrenaline reduces local bleeding, if sufficient time (10–15 minutes) is allowed to elapse between injection and incision. Local anaesthetics containing adrenaline must never be used near end-arteries, such as digits, nose, penis, or pinna; nor for intravenous regional anaesthesia. Adrenaline should be used with caution in patients with thyrotoxicosis, hypertension, ischaemic heart disease, peripheral vascular disease, or phaeochromocytoma. It can safely be given to patients taking monoamine oxidase inhibitors, but should be used with caution in those taking tricyclic antidepressants. Adrenaline should be avoided in patients receiving halothane anaesthesia, as the myocardium is sensitized to catecholamines and cardiac arrhythmias are likely, especially in the presence of hypercapnia. Felypressin is a synthetic polypeptide related to vasopressin which is added to some local anaesthetics as a vasoconstrictor (usually 0.03 units/ml). It is less toxic than adrenaline, and may be used when adrenaline is contraindicated. Methylhydroxybenzoate (methylparaben) is used as a preservative in multidose vials of some local anaesthetics. It is non-toxic in small concentrations, but allergic reactions have been reported after its administration. It should not be used for intravenous regional anaesthesia.

Further reading

Covino, B. G. (1986). Pharmacology of local anaesthetic agents. *British Journal of Anaesthesia*, **58**, 701–16.

Tucker, G. J. (1986). Pharmacokinetics of local anaesthetics. *British Journal of Anaesthesia*, **58**, 717–31.

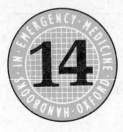

CHAPTER 14

Problems encountered during local anaesthesia

Key points in problems during local anaesthesia

- Never start an operation until adequate anaesthesia has been obtained
- Never exceed the maximum dose or volume of local anaesthetic when supplementing a failed block
- Everyone using local anaesthetics must be competent at managing the possible toxic effects
- Problems may be minimized by meticulous attention to technique

Failed nerve blocks

Always believe a patient who says that the local anaesthetic is not working. She or he is likely to be correct even if the nerve block technique appeared to be perfect. Good surface analgesia may occur without anaesthesia of deeper tissues. A nerve block may fail for a number of reasons.

Incorrect timing

Not enough time may be given for the local anaesthetic to work. This occurs more commonly in major nerve blocks, which may take up to 40 minutes to work, or when the doctor is in a hurry to complete a procedure. The local anaesthetic effect may wear off too quickly. This may happen with short acting blocks such as infiltration techniques. In this situation it is worthwhile considering the use of adrenaline with the local anaesthetic to prolong the duration of anaesthesia.

Incorrect site of injection

Local anaesthetic may be injected too far away from the nerve. It is important to ensure that the patient is comfortable so that the landmarks are easily identified. It is more difficult to find the correct landmarks in obese patients.

Incorrect dose of local anaesthetic

Insufficient local anaesthetic may be used to block the nerve. For example in certain blocks, such as the femoral nerve block, the volume of local anaesthetic used may be critical.

Management of a failed nerve block

If a nerve block fails and an operative procedure has to be performed, other techniques can be used. Check that sufficient time has elapsed for the particular nerve block to work, and never exceed the maximum dose or volume of local anaesthetic.

If there has been no altered sensation then the local anaesthetic has probably been injected too far away from the nerve. Occasionally in major nerve blocks total absence of block may occur if too small a volume of local anaesthetic has been used. Identify the necessary landmarks and confirm the correct site for injection. Repeat the block using half the initial dose, having first ensured that neither the maximum dose nor the maximum volume has been exceeded.

Patchy anaesthesia is unacceptable for operative procedures. It occurs when insufficient local anaesthetic penetrates the nerve, because of either inadequate dosage or incorrect siting of the injection. It is also a sign of a block wearing off. Repeat the block using half the initial dose, ensuring that this does not exceed the maximum dose or the maximum volume.

If the block is still unsuccessful consider using a more proximal nerve block, such as an ulnar nerve block at the wrist instead of a digital nerve block at the base of the little finger.

Local anaesthesia may be supplemented with Entonox for short procedures, such as the uncomplicated reduction of a dislocation. In other situations it may be better to abandon the local anaesthetic technique and obtain controlled conditions by using a general anaesthetic.

Complications of local anaesthesia

Acute systemic toxicity

Acute systemic toxicity occurs when the local anaesthetic blood concentration exceeds the toxic level. The blood concentration is determined by the rates of vascular absorption, tissue redistribution, metabolism, and excretion. Thus patients at the extremes of age or with renal or hepatic impairment are more at risk of systemic toxicity. The rate of absorption is influenced by the site of injection. An intercostal block produces more than three times the maximum plasma concentration of lignocaine than is seen after local infiltration. Absorption of local anaesthetic increases as follows: femoral block < sciatic block < brachial plexus block < epidural < caudal < intercostal block. Rapid absorption may also occur with local infiltration or topical anaesthesia of the respiratory tract. The addition of adrenaline to the local anaesthetic reduces the peak blood concentration, but the degree of reduction depends on the site of injection and the type of local anaesthetic. Adrenaline produces about a 50 per cent decrease in peak blood concentrations of lignocaine given by subcutaneous infiltration, but only a 20–30 per cent decrease with brachial plexus or intercostal blocks. Adrenaline decreases the peak blood concentrations of bupivacaine much less than lignocaine.

Acute systemic toxicity is most commonly caused by accidental intravascular injection. A dose much less than the recommended maximum dose may produce a toxic reaction by this route. Systemic toxicity may occur when an overdose of the local anaesthetic is given through ignorance or miscalculation of the maximum dose.

The main toxic effects are on the central nervous system and the cardiovascular system. The latter appears to be more resistant to the local anaesthetic's effects than the former. It should not be assumed that the patient will demonstrate all the stages of toxicity. There may be immediate convulsions; or the first sign may not become apparent until 1 to 2 minutes after completion of the injection. Maximum plasma levels develop within about 10 to 25 minutes after an uneventful procedure. Patients should be observed for at least 30 minutes after nerve blocks when doses approaching the recommended maximum level are used.

Central nervous system signs and symptoms

Mild toxicity produces signs of a central nervous stimulation due to depression of the inhibitory centres, which progresses to central nervous depression as the severity increases. Numbness of the tongue and mouth (a local effect due to local anaesthetic leaving the vascular space and affecting sensory nerve endings) may occur, followed by lightheadedness, tinnitus, visual disturbance, and slurring of speech. With more severe reactions there may be muscle twitching, confusion, convulsion, coma, and apnoea.

Early signs of toxicity can be identified if the doctor maintains a conversation with the patient during the injection. Muscle twitching may be caused by shivering due to cold or nervousness. Irrational behaviour may have to be distinguished from hysterical or neurotic reactions. Fainting may also occur during local anaesthetic procedures. Cardiovascular signs may help in making the correct diagnosis.

Cardiovascular signs and symptoms

The initial signs of toxicity are hypertension and tachycardia related to blocking of central nervous system inhibitory centres. Local anaesthetics have a direct action on cardiac muscle. This produces a negative inotropic effect, with moderate hypotension and a decrease in cardiac output. There may be vasodilatation due to a direct effect on vascular smooth muscle. Severe hypotension may follow. Slowing of the conducting system causes sinus bradycardia and conduction defects. Ventricular arrhythmias and cardiac arrest may occur, especially with bupivacaine.

Treatment of toxicity

Stop injecting the local anaesthetic immediately something appears to be wrong. The basic 'airway, breathing, circulation' principles of resuscitation apply in all cases. Toxic reactions are potentiated by hypoxaemia and acidosis. Oxygen should be given and intravenous access should be established. Record pulse rate, blood pressure, respiratory rate, and consciousness level, and monitor the electrocardiogram.

Central nervous system toxicity

Convulsions should be treated rapidly. The following anticonvulsants may be used (approximate adult dose indicated):

- Diazemuls 5–10 mg IV slowly (0.1–0.2 mg/kg)
- Thiopentone 50 mg increments IV slowly (1–2 mg/kg)

Diazemuls is the drug of choice for those without anaesthetic training. Thiopentone is preferable because of its rapid effect and short duration of action, but it can cause marked ventilatory depression and hypotension, and must only be given by those experienced in its use. The convulsions will not last longer than a few minutes, and seldom recur once the anticonvulsant has been effective, except in a massive overdose. Thus once thiopentone has worn off the patient should be awake and rational within a few minutes. If Diazemuls is used the patient may take longer to wake up.

Cardiovascular toxicity: hypotension

Raise the foot of the trolley. If the systolic blood pressure is less than 90 mmHg in an adult give 500 ml of colloid solution. This may be repeated if the hypotension persists. In a child, treat if the systolic pressure falls below 70 mm Hg, giving an initial bolus of 20 ml/kg of colloid solution.

Cardiovascular toxicity: cardiac arrhythmias

The arrhythmias may resolve spontaneously. Treatment should only be given if a severe reduction in the cardiac output occurs. Atropine may help treat bradycardia and severe hypotension. Cardiac pacing may be required for complete heart block. Bretylium may be successful in treating ventricular fibrillation unresponsive to DC shock. Cardiotoxicity is more severe with bupivacaine. Successful cardiac resuscitation after accidental intravenous administration may take over 30 minutes. Correct any hyperkalaemia, which potentiates the toxic effects.

Serious local anaesthetic toxicity is usually preventable if emphasis is placed on a scrupulous technique and a knowledge of the maximum safe dose for every patient (Tables 12.1, 12.2, p. 274).

Allergic reactions

Severe allergic reactions to local anaesthetic agents are rare. Symptoms must be distinguished from those due to anxiety or simple fainting. Systemic toxicity due to the local anaesthetic or added vasoconstrictors must also be considered.

Local anaesthetics of the ester group, such as cocaine, procaine, or amethocaine more commonly produce allergic reactions than those from the amide group, such as lignocaine or bupivacaine. The ester-derived agents are used much less commonly than the amides. Patients who are allergic to one ester are likely to show cross-sensitivity with the whole group, but not with the amides. Patients who are allergic to an amide may not react to different amides. Testing for hypersensitivity with small doses has not proved reliable.

Dental practice has provided the most reports of adverse reactions to local anaesthetics. Persisting pain at the injection site and local tissue swelling are most common. The latter may reflect a type IV hypersensitivity (contact allergy) or sensitive tissues. The possibility that the trauma of injection has triggered angio-oedema in a patient with C1 esterase inhibitor deficiency should be considered.

Multidose vials of local anaesthetic may contain the preservative methyl hydroxybenzoate (methylparaben) which can cause allergic reactions. It may be the cause of presumed sensitivity to local anaesthetics or other drug preparations. Local anaesthetic from multidose vials should never be used for intravenous regional anaesthesia.

Local infection

Infection may be introduced from contaminated equipment or may arise as a result of local spread from the patient.

Haematoma and bruising

Extra care should be taken when inserting a needle close to a vessel. Bleeding can usually be controlled by direct pressure.

Needle breakage

This most commonly occurs where the needle joins the hub. It is important to use a needle of sufficient length and never to advance it right up to the hub. Redirecting the needle may also cause it to break. Always withdraw the needle to just below the skin before repositioning, so that minimal leverage is applied to the shaft.

Nerve damage

Division, compression, stretching, or ischaemic damage to nerves may occur during a local anaesthetic procedure or subsequent surgery. Traumatic damage may be reduced by using a needle with a short bevel or pencil point. Eliciting paraesthesia may increase the risk of nerve damage and should not be used routinely. Paraesthesia may occur during the routine technique. If paraesthesia is felt, the needle should be withdrawn slightly before injection, since intra-neural injection could cause permanent nerve damage. Injecting slowly reduces the risk of nerve damage. Stretching or compression of the nerve may occur because of incorrect positioning of the patient or poor use of equipment such as tourniquets, arm rests, or retractors.

Ischaemia and necrosis

Necrosis and gangrene may occur after the incorrect use of a vasoconstrictor around an end-artery. It is advisable to store all local anaesthetic with adrenaline in locked cupboards, separately from the routine plain preparations.

Management of accidental injection of adrenaline around an end-artery
The patient should be admitted for observation and the consultant should be informed. Analgesia may be required. Consider the use of anticoagulation with heparin, vaso-dilators, and sympathetic blockade.

Unintentional blockage of additional nerves

This may occur with nerve blocks around the eye, where local anaesthetic leaking through to the optic nerve may cause temporary blindness. Large volume injections into the femoral canal may block the whole lumbar plexus.

Retrograde arterial spread

This may follow high pressure injections with dental syringes in the head region. Convulsions may occur.

Reactions to vasoconstrictors

Serious reactions due to the use of adrenaline in local anaesthesia are rare, and occur more commonly if high concentrations are used. The maximum dose is 500 μg in adults. Intraosseous injections of small volumes of adrenaline at 1:80 000 during dental procedures have been associated with symptoms such as apprehension, restlessness, sweating, tachycardia, palpitations, and tightness in the chest. Inadvertent intravascular injection may also cause serious complications, especially tachycardia, dysrhythmias, and hypertension.

Treatment of adrenaline toxicity

This will be governed by the patient's haemodynamic state. Monitor the pulse rate, blood pressure, and electrocardiogram. Give oxygen by face mask. Sublingual glyceryl trinitrate should be given (by tablet or spray) to patients who develop angina. Patients with a tachycardia should be admitted for observation, until it settles. Beta-adrenergic blocking drugs may be useful for persistent tachycardia. Infusion of a short acting vasodilator such as glyceryl trinitrate may control raised arterial blood pressure and would require direct arterial pressure monitoring.

Psychogenic reactions

Fear and pain can cause reflex vasomotor disturbances. Young adults may get vagal overactivity, causing severe bradycardia. Pallor, nausea, sweating, and hypotension causing syncope may also occur. These reactions are more common if the patient is sitting upright. Cerebral hypoxaemia with loss of consciousness and tremors or convulsions may occur before the patient can be laid flat. The patient should be placed in the coma position and given oxygen. Sustained bradycardia (heart rate < 45/min) may require a slow intravenous injection of 0.5 mg atropine.

Prolonged blockage

This is a rare, idiosyncratic event.

Methaemoglobinaemia

Prilocaine may cause methaemoglobinaemia if doses in excess of 7 mg/kg are used. Its metabolite *o*-toluidine causes oxidation of haemoglobin. The patient may complain of a headache and may be dyspnoeic or centrally cyanosed. Pulse oximetry readings will be inaccurate, overestimating the arterial oxygen saturation. Methaemoglobinaemia may be confirmed by laboratory investigation.

Treatment of methaemoglobinaemia

Oxygen should be administered if the patient is dyspnoeic. Methylene blue 1 per cent solution should be given intravenously in a dose of 1–4 mg/kg over 5 minutes. This may be repeated if necessary. Extravasation of the drug should be avoided, because subcutaneous injection causes necrotic abscesses.

Further reading

Reynolds, F. (1987). Adverse effects of local anaesthetics. *British Journal of Anaesthesia*, **59**, 78–95.

Scott, D. B. (1986). Toxic effects of local anaesthetic agents on the central nervous system. *British Journal of Anaesthesia*, **58**, 732–5.

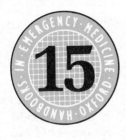

CHAPTER 15

Local anaesthetic nerve blocks: local infiltration of the skin

Local infiltration of the skin (Fig. 15.1)

Indications

- Suturing lacerations
- Minor surgical procedures (e.g. excision of cyst)
- Supplementing a nerve block
- Cleaning and debriding wounds
- Venous cannulation, using 1 per cent lignocaine administered subcutaneously is less painful than with 18, 20 or 22 Guage cannulae alone.

Special contraindications

None.

Anatomy

Distal nerve endings and filaments are blocked at the site of infiltration.

Landmarks

Area to be anaesthetized and local blood vessels to be avoided during injection.

Positioning

The patient should rest comfortably, allowing optimal exposure of the operative site.

Dosage

Up to 20 ml of 1 per cent lignocaine or 40 ml of 0.5 per cent lignocaine with or without adrenaline. Larger doses of local anaesthetic may be used with adrenaline (Tables 12.1, 12.2, p. 274).

Equipment

23 gauge $\times$ 1.25 inch (0.6 $\times$ 30 mm) needle and 2, 5, 10, or 20 ml syringe.

Technique

Inject local anaesthetic around the area to be treated. If a second puncture is required always reintroduce the needle through previously anaesthetized skin. The patient should only feel one injection.

Onset and duration

Onset: 2–3 minutes.
Duration: up to 45 minutes, depending on whether a vaso-constrictor is used.

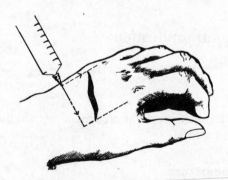

Fig. 15.1 • Local infiltration of the skin.

Comments

- Never use a vasoconstrictor around end arteries such as those of the digits, ear, nose, or penis.
- For most wounds requiring suturing under an infiltration block it is helpful to avoid injecting the local anaesthetic directly along the wound margin, as this reduces distortion of the wound edges and aids good skin apposition.
- Injection into the wound edge may be indicated for simple wounds in children, since this approach is less painful. However, it may introduce infection, and should not be used if the wound is contaminated.
- When the nerve supply to an area comes from one side this alone need be blocked – for example, the dorsum of the hand.
- When using large volumes of local anaesthetic ensure that the maximum dose for local anaesthetic and adrenaline is not exceeded.

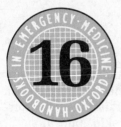

CHAPTER 16

Nerve blocks of the upper limb

Brachial plexus block

Indications

Brachial plexus block can be used for surgery or manipulation of a fracture and/or dislocation in one upper limb (bilateral block is not recommended). It can also be used to produce vasodilatation of the upper limb after intra-arterial injection of irritants. It is useful when either the use of a tourniquet is contraindicated or it would need releasing during the procedure. It provides better postoperative pain relief than IVRA. There are three approaches to the brachial plexus: axillary, subclavian perivascular, and interscalene. Plasma local anaesthetic levels are similar with all three techniques.

The effect of a block at each level can be predicted from a knowledge of the anatomy. Axillary block can be used for procedures below the elbow. Subclavian perivascular or interscalene block can be used for procedures which also involve the upper arm and shoulder. Each method has advantages and disadvantages. The axillary approach is the safest and that most commonly used in the A & E department. The dose of local anaesthetic required is large, and the potential for adverse effects exists. Patients should have a full preoperative assessment and be fasted for 4 hours before the procedure.

Special contraindications

- Inability to abduct the arm or lymphangitis of the arm contraindicate the axillary technique

- Phrenic or recurrent laryngeal nerve paralysis on the contralateral side, pneumothorax on the contralateral side, and severe respiratory disease contraindicate the subclavian perivascular or interscalene approaches
- In the A & E department subclavian perivascular and interscalene block are not appropriate for use in children, and axillary block should probably be avoided in children under 10 years old

Anatomy

The brachial plexus supplies the upper limb. Its roots are formed from the anterior primary rami of C5, C6, C7, C8, and T1, which emerge from the cervical spine between the anterior and middle scalene muscles in the neck. The roots unite in the posterior triangle of the neck to form three trunks: C5 and C6 form the upper trunk, C7 forms the middle trunk, and C8 and T1 form the lower trunk. The trunks pass over the first rib, lying on top of each other, superior to the subclavian artery, and behind the mid-point of the clavicle, where each trunk divides into an anterior and a posterior division. The divisions form cords which pass into the axilla, and are named according to their arrangement around the axillary artery.

The lateral cord is formed by the anterior divisions of the upper and middle trunks; it gives rise to the musculocutaneous nerve (which terminates as the lateral cutaneous nerve of the forearm) and the lateral head of the median nerve. The medial cord is a continuation of the anterior division of the lower trunk. Its largest branch is the ulnar nerve; however, it also gives rise to the medial head of the median nerve and the medial cutaneous nerves of the arm and forearm. The three posterior divisions form the posterior cord, which gives rise to the axillary nerve (which terminates as the upper lateral cutaneous nerve of the arm) and the radial nerve (which branches in the axilla to give the posterior cutaneous nerve of the arm, and branches in the arm to give the lower lateral cutaneous nerve of the arm and the posterior cutaneous nerve of the forearm). Figure 16.1 shows a simplified diagram of the innervation of the upper limb; however, there is much overlap between the various nerves. The skin of the axilla is supplied by the inter-

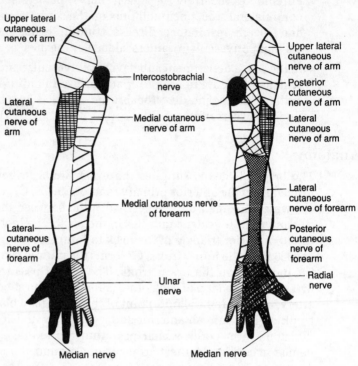

Fig. 16.1 • Cutaneous innervation of the upper limb.

Table 16.1 • Calculation of the volume of the brachial perivascular space

Age (years)	Volume (ml)
1–4	Height (inches)/5
5–8	Height (inches)/4
9–16	Height (inches)/3
> 16	Height (inches)/2

The volume of local anaesthetic should be calculated, and then the dose should be checked to ensure that it is below toxic limits. The volume may be slightly reduced for debilitated patients.

costobrachial nerve, which is formed by the lateral branches of the second, and sometimes the third, intercostal nerves.

The prevertebral fascia envelops the brachial plexus from the level of the cervical vertebrae to the distal axilla, forming a subclavian perivascular space which is in continuity with the axillary perivascular space. Once this space has been entered by a needle, only a single injection is necessary for anaesthesia of the brachial plexus. The extent of the block is dependent upon the volume of local anaesthetic injected and the level at which the needle is placed. The volume of the space can be calculated (Table 16.1).

Axillary block

Landmark

Pulsation of the axillary artery high in the axilla, between the pectoralis major and the latissimus dorsi muscles.

Positioning

The patient is supine, with the arm abducted to 90° and the elbow flexed. The arm should be relaxed and comfortably placed next to the head; not under the head, as this may make the axillary artery less discernible. Venous access should be established in the contralateral arm, ECG, pulse oximetry, and blood pressure monitoring should be instituted prior to the procedure.

Dosage

A dose of 40 ml of 1 per cent lignocaine with 1:200 000 adrenaline or 40 ml of 0.375 per cent plain bupivacaine (for a longer effect) in a healthy adult; for children see Table 16.1.

Equipment

- Resuscitation equipment
- A short bevelled or pencil point 23 gauge × 3.5 inch (0.6 × 84 mm) needle; cutting needles must not be used because of the risk of nerve damage.
- An extension for the needle to allow remote injection
- Two 20 ml syringes

Technique

1. Palpate the axillary artery as high in the axilla as possible. If it is not easily felt, the arm may be too abducted or

the patient may be tense; adjust the position of the arm and reassure the patient.

2. Warn the patient that he or she may experience paraesthesia. Insert the needle, with the extension attached, superior to the artery and as close to it as possible, at an angle of 30°–40° to the skin. Pulsation of the needle confirms proximity to the artery. Attempts to illicit paraesthesia may result in nerve damage, but if paraesthesia occurs, this confirms proximity to the plexus. A click may be felt as the needle enters the fascial sheath around the brachial plexus; but this is not a reliable sign of good needle placement. If aspiration shows that the needle has entered the axillary artery, the needle should be advanced until repeated aspiration demonstrates that it has just left the artery by piercing its posterior wall; the needle will now be in the posterior part of the sheath around the brachial plexus. If PNS is used, then movement of the wrist or fingers should be sought. Elbow flexion alone is associated with a significant incidence of failed block.

3. Once the needle is inside the brachial plexus sheath apply pressure with the thumb, distal to the point of injection to encourage proximal spread of local anaesthetic. Aspirate again to confirm that the needle is not intravascular. Slowly inject 38 ml of the local anaesthetic via the extension, monitoring the patient carefully. Once local anaesthetic has been injected, repositioning of the needle should not be attempted, as partial anaesthesia may obtund the pain of perineural injection and nerve damage may occur.

4. After injection partly withdraw the needle and inject the remaining 2 ml subcutaneously to block the intercostobrachial nerve. Remove the needle, press over the injection site, and adduct the arm to the side; this last manœuvre moves the head of the humerus and encourages proximal spread of local anaesthetic.

5. Wait 30 minutes before testing the adequacy of the block. Axillary and intercostobrachial block should produce anaesthesia sufficient for procedures below the elbow, and will usually permit pain free application of a tourni-

quet. It cannot be relied upon for procedures in the upper arm or shoulder.

6. The extent of block of the brachial plexus is dependent upon the volume of local anaesthetic injected. The musculocutaneous and axillary nerves leave the brachial plexus at a high level, and can only be consistently blocked, in an adult, if at least 40 ml of local anaesthetic are placed in the neurovascular sheath. If small volumes, such as 20–30 ml, are used, these branches are commonly missed, and sensation is preserved over the lateral aspect of the upper arm and forearm; surgery is not possible in this area, and tourniquet pain is a potential problem. Combined radial and lateral cutaneous nerve of forearm block may be performed to supplement the axillary block, using 1 per cent lignocaine with 1:200 000 adrenaline, as long as the total dose of local anaesthetic and adrenaline does not exceed toxic amounts (p. 323).

Onset and duration

Onset: lignocaine 30 minutes, bupivacaine 30–45 minutes. The patient will often lose extension at the elbow first.
Duration: lignocaine 4–6 hours, bupivacaine 6–12 hours. It is important to warn the patient, and staff, to protect the anaesthetized limb until sensation returns. Hyperextension of joints must be avoided, and the arm should be supported in a sling.

Comments

- If larger volumes (50–60 ml) are used for axillary block, the cervical plexus will also be affected, as it travels in the same space, but at a higher level.

- Although the transarterial approach is a recognized technique, its use should be discouraged; it may result in haematoma formation, and bleeding from the artery dilutes the local anaesthetic. Injection above and below the axillary artery was once advocated; however, this is unnecessary once the concept of the neurovascular sheath is understood; repeated injection increases the risk of arterial puncture and nerve damage.

Subclavian perivascular block (Fig. 16.2)

Landmarks

The sternomastoid muscle and the pulsation of the sub-clavian artery at the base of the interscalene groove.

Positioning

The patient is supine, with one pillow under the head, which is turned away from the side to be blocked. The patient is asked to keep the arm by the side and reach towards the knee to depress the shoulder and clavicle. Venous access should be established in the contralateral arm, ECG, transcutaneous oxygen saturation, and blood pressure monitoring should be instituted prior to the procedure.

Dosage

A dose of 40 ml of 1 per cent lignocaine with 1:200 000 adrenaline or 40 ml of 0.375 per cent plain bupivacaine (for a longer effect) in an adult.

Equipment

- Resuscitation equipment
- 23 gauge × 3.5 inch (0.6 × 84 mm) short bevelled or pencil point needle; cutting needles should not be used for plexus anaesthesia
- Extension to allow remote injection
- Two 20 ml syringes

Technique

1. Palpate the lateral edge of the sternomastoid muscle just above the clavicle; ask the patient to lift the head to make this more prominent. Roll the index finger laterally over the belly of the anterior scalene muscle (this can be made more prominent by asking the patient to take a deep breath) until the interscalene groove is palpable. Run the finger along the groove towards the clavicle until the pulsation of the subclavian artery is felt as it emerges between the scalene muscles.

2. With a finger still on the artery, warn the patient that he or she will feel paraesthesia. Insert the needle, with an extension attached, above this point, and aim it caudally in a direction parallel to the scalene muscles until the patient describes paraesthesia going below the elbow (Fig. 16.2). Paraesthesia in the shoulder or over the chest wall indicates stimulation of the suprascapular or long thoracic nerves *outside* the neurovascular sheath, and the needle should be withdrawn and redirected. Paraesthesia usually occurs before the first rib is contacted. If a PNS is used, elbow movement should be sought.

3. Once paraesthesiae have been elicited, aspirate to confirm that the needle is extravascular, and slowly inject the local anaesthetic, observing the patient.

4. If it is possible to abduct the arm, inject 2–3 ml of local anaesthetic subcutaneously over the axillary artery to block the intercostobrachial nerve.

5. Wait 15 minutes before checking the adequacy of the block. Subclavian perivascular block will produce anaesthesia for procedures on the shoulder or arm, and supplementation by intercostobrachial block will allow pain free tourniquet application.

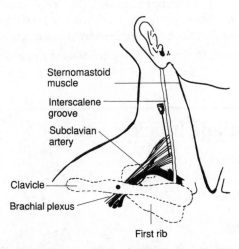

Fig. 16.2 • Subclavian perivascular brachial plexus block.

Onset and duration

Onset: 15–30 minutes; the patient often loses shoulder movement first.

Duration: lignocaine 4–6 hours, bupivacaine 6–12 hours. It is important to warn the patient, and staff, to protect the blocked limb until sensation returns. Hyperextension of joints must be avoided, and the arm should be supported in a sling.

Comments

- Pneumothorax may occur, especially if the needle is directed too medially. Patients should be admitted to hospital for 24 hours after the block, as the signs of pneumothorax may be delayed.

- Phrenic nerve paralysis occurs in a third of cases and laryngeal nerve block, cervical plexus block, and sympathetic block are common.

- The subclavian artery may be punctured, but this does not usually cause problems.

- As the technique relies on eliciting paraesthesia, nerve damage is theoretically possible.

- The subclavian perivascular technique has a useful place in the provision of anaesthesia in the upper limb, particularly for manipulation of a dislocated shoulder. However, it has more potential risks than the axillary approach, and should only be performed by those experienced in its use.

- Its use in the A & E department is limited by the necessity to admit patients for 24 hours' observation afterwards.

Interscalene block (Fig. 16.3)

Landmarks

Sternomastoid muscle, interscalene groove, and cricoid cartilage.

Positioning

The patient is supine, with one pillow under the head, which is turned away from the side to be blocked. Venous

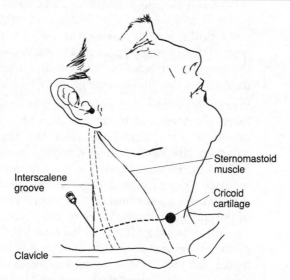

Fig. 16.3 • Interscalene brachial plexus block.

access should be established in the contralateral arm ECG, oxygen saturation, and blood pressure monitoring should be instituted prior to the procedure.

Dosage

A dose of 40 ml of 1 per cent lignocaine with 1:200 000 adrenaline or 40 ml of 0.375 per cent plain bupivacaine (for a longer effect) in an adult.

Equipment

- Resuscitation equipment
- Short bevelled or pencil point 23 gauge × 3.5 inch (0.6 × 84 mm) needle; cutting needles must not be used because of the risk of nerve damage.
- Extension for needle to allow remote injection
- Two 20 ml syringes

Technique

1. Palpate the lateral edge of the sternomastoid muscle just above the clavicle; ask the patient to lift the head to make

this more prominent. Roll the index finger laterally over the belly of the anterior scalene muscle (this can be made more prominent by asking the patient to take a deep breath) until the interscalene groove is palpable. Palpate the cricoid cartilage, and draw a line laterally from it to impinge on the interscalene groove (see Fig. 16.3).

2. Warn the patient that he or she may feel paraesthesia. Insert the needle with an extension into the interscalene groove at the point level with the cricoid cartilage. Advance the needle in a direction which is perpendicular to the skin in all planes. The needle is moving medially, dorsally, and slightly caudally. Advance the needle until paraesthesia is felt or the transverse process of the cervical vertebra is contacted (usually less than 2.5 cm from the skin). If a PNS is being used, shoulder and elbow movement should be sought. It is important not to direct the needle too horizontally, as it may not be stopped by the transverse process, but may enter the vertebral artery, the epidural space, or a dural cuff, with potentially dangerous results.

3. Aspirate to ensure that the needle is not intravascular or in a dural sleeve (failure to aspirate cerebrospinal fluid cannot guarantee that the needle is not subarachnoid). Apply pressure with one finger proximal to the needle insertion to encourage caudal spread of local anaesthetic. Slowly inject the local anaesthetic, and observe the patient carefully.

4. If it is possible to abduct the arm, inject 2–3 ml of local anaesthetic subcutaneously over the axillary artery to block the intercostobrachial nerve.

5. Wait 15 minutes before checking the adequacy of the block. Interscalene block will produce anaesthesia for procedures on the shoulder or arm, and supplementation by intercostobrachial block will allow pain free tourniquet application.

6. Block of the ulnar nerve may be delayed or absent after interscalene block, especially if less than 40 ml of local anaesthetic is used. Sensation will be preserved in the ulnar border of the hand and the little and ring fingers. Ulnar nerve block may be performed to supplement inter-

scalene block, using 1 per cent lignocaine with 1:200 000 adrenaline, as long as the total dose of local anaesthetic does not exceed toxic amounts (p. 320).

Onset and duration

Onset: 15–30 minutes; the patient often loses shoulder movement first.

Duration: lignocaine 4–6 hours, bupivacaine 6–12 hours. It is important to warn the patient, and staff, to protect the blocked limb until sensation returns. Hyperextension of joints must be avoided, and the arm should be supported in a sling.

Comments

- The risk of pneumothorax is less after the interscalene approach than with the subclavian perivascular technique. The potential for serious adverse effects is greatest with the interscalene block. Its use in the A & E department should be limited. Only those experienced in the technique and competent to manage adverse effects should use this block.

- Adverse effects tend to be immediate. If the local anaesthetic is injected into the vertebral artery a serious toxic reaction will result.

- The potential for a very high epidural or 'total spinal' injection also exists.

- Recurrent laryngeal nerve, phrenic nerve, sympathetic, and cervical plexus block is common.

Intravenous regional anaesthesia (IVRA) of the upper limb

Indications

IVRA (Bier's block) is widely used in A & E departments to provide anaesthesia and muscle relaxation for minor surgery or fracture reduction below the elbow in one arm. IVRA is superior to infiltration of the fracture site for reduction of Colles' fracture (Cobb and Houghton 1985). IVRA is a simple, reliable technique. There is always a risk of a toxic reaction, because a large dose of local anaesthetic is required. A full preoperative assessment should be carried out before IVRA, and patients should be fasted for 4 hours. Only medical staff competent to deal with a severe toxic reaction to the local anaesthetic should perform IVRA. Two trained members of staff must be present at all times.

Special contraindications

- Procedures to be performed on both upper limbs, as the amount of local anaesthetic needed for bilateral IVRA would exceed the toxic dose.
- Surgery which will take more than 30 minutes, as tourniquet pain will be a problem.
- Surgery where the tourniquet may need releasing, such as operations on blood vessels.
- Severe hypertension, obesity or Monckeberg's calcinosis, which may lead to leakage of local anaesthetic under the tourniquet.
- Sickle cell disease or trait.
- Children under 7 years old.
- Infection in the limb.
- Severe peripheral vascular disease.
- Use with caution in patients with epilepsy.

Anatomy

Local anaesthetic diffuses out of the vascular system to act on peripheral nerves. Small veins are valveless and communicate with venules in nerve trunks. Positron emission tomography shows that local anaesthetic is rapidly taken up by nerve trunks within 2–4 minutes after injection. Once the tourniquet is released the local anaesthetic leaves the neural tissue rapidly.

Positioning

The patient should be supine on a tipping trolley.

Dosage

A dose of 0.5 per cent *plain* prilocaine, from a single dose vial without preservative, is the drug of choice (Table 16.2);

Table 16.2 • Volume of 0.5% plain* prilocaine for IVRA

Adult	40 ml
Very thin/elderly/debilitated patients	30 ml
Adolescent aged 14–17 years	30 ml
Child aged 11–13 years	20 ml
Child aged 7–10 years	15 ml

* Solutions with adrenaline or preservative must not be used.

it is the least toxic agent, and has been associated with the fewest reports of adverse effects (Wallace *et al.* 1982). There is no advantage to the use of lignocaine. Bupivacaine is not recommended for IVRA, because severe toxic reactions, including some deaths, have occurred during its use.

Equipment

- Resuscitation equipment.
- Pressure compensated tourniquet with a 15 cm cuff for adults and a single cuff which is two-thirds the length of the upper arm for children. Deaths have occurred during IVRA as a result of accidental deflation of the cuff. The tourniquet must be reliable, free from leaks, and regularly serviced. Ordinary blood pressure cuffs should not be used.
- An Esmarch bandage or an inflatable splint is sometimes needed (but is often too painful to use after trauma).
- A small winged needle or cannula.

Technique

The Casualty Surgeons' Association published guidelines (1983) on the use of IVRA in A & E departments. Venous access should be established in the contralateral arm before commencing the procedure. ECG, pulse oximetry, and blood pressure monitoring should be used.

1. Fully expose the arm to be operated on and place the tourniquet high on the upper arm over some padding. Site a small cannula in a vein on the dorsum of the hand on the operative side. Palpate the radial pulse.

2. Elevate the arm above the level of the heart for 3 minutes to exsanguinate the limb (pressure over the brachial

artery may help). An Esmarch bandage or inflatable splint may be used to aid exsanguination. This is only possible if the arm is not painful. Elevate the tourniquet to 300 mm Hg or 100 mm Hg more than the preoperative systolic blood pressure (which ever is greater). Place the arm comfortably on a pillow. Check that the tourniquet is tight and not leaking, and that the radial pulse is no longer palpable. Record the time of application of the tourniquet.

3. Slowly inject the required volume of 0.5 per cent plain prilocaine (Table 16.2) into the cannula in the isolated limb, which will become mottled after injection. If the hand is the site of operation ask an assistant to squeeze the forearm tightly during injection, aiming to direct more local anaesthetic peripherally. Record the time of injection.

4. After 5 minutes test for anaesthesia. If the block is incomplete inject 10–15 ml normal saline into the cannula to flush more prilocaine peripherally.

5. Constant observation of the tourniquet pressure must be maintained. The cuff must remain elevated for at least 20 minutes, even if surgery is completed in a shorter time. After 20 minutes deflate the tourniquet and record the time. The limb will feel warm and tingly, and will usually flush. Sensation can return quickly, and postoperative analgesia may be needed.

6. Observe the patient carefully for at least 2 hours after the procedure and record routine observations.

7. Check the circulation of the limb before discharging the patient.

Onset and duration

Onset: 2–5 minutes.
Duration: 2–80 minutes after release of the tourniquet (mean duration approximately 20 minutes). Surgery cannot be resumed after the cuff has been deflated. as sensation can return quickly.

Comments

- Vasoconstrictors must never be used for IVRA.

- After tourniquet release entry of local anaesthetic into the circulation is biphasic. Longer cuff application delays wash out of local anaesthetic and reduces peak plasma concentrations. Studies using lignocaine have demonstrated that 20–30 per cent of the injected dose entered the systemic circulation during the first minute after deflation of a cuff (which had been inflated for 10 minutes), and the remaining lignocaine emerged more slowly; 50 per cent of the initial dose persisted in the arm 30 minutes after tourniquet release (Tucker and Boas 1971). Hence the need to observe patients closely after IVRA.

- Even a tight tourniquet will not totally preclude entry of local anaesthetic into the general circulation. Some drug passes via the interosseous route, and some leaks under the tourniquet. Plasma local anaesthetic concentrations can be reduced by good exsanguination, meticulous checking of tourniquet pressure, slow injection, and the use of distal rather than antecubital veins.

- Tourniquet pain can be a problem during IVRA. The use of a double cuff has been advocated to reduce this. A second cuff is inflated distal to the first cuff, over an area of anaesthetized skin; the initial cuff is then deflated. The use of a double cuff increases the risk of unintentional tourniquet deflation, and should be avoided if possible.

- Reactive swelling can occur after IVRA. A back slab should be applied to immobilize fractures, and completed only when any swelling has subsided.

- Local anaesthetic toxicity may occur after accidental or intentional tourniquet release. If accidental tourniquet deflation occurs, reinflate the cuff if possible, or apply an ordinary cuff proximally. Monitor the patient and prepare to treat any local anaesthetic toxicity (see p. 292).

- If IVRA fails to give adequate anaesthesia no further local anaesthetic should be given and the patient should usually receive general anaesthesia.

- At least seven deaths, two cardiopulmonary arrests, and ten cases of convulsions have been reported after IVRA. Although the technique is valuable, it should be used with respect, by doctors proficient in resuscitation.

Ulnar nerve block at the elbow (Fig. 16.4)

Indications

Minor surgery in the area of innervation of the ulnar nerve and to supplement inadequate brachial plexus block.

Special contraindications

None.

Anatomy

The ulnar nerve arises from the C7, C8, and T1 nerve roots, and is formed from the medial cord of the brachial plexus. It lies medial to the axillary and brachial artery until it reaches the middle of the humerus, when it pierces the intermuscular septum to enter the extensor compartment, and then descends on the anterior aspect of triceps. At the elbow it passes behind the medial epicondyle to enter the forearm between the two heads of flexor carpi ulnaris.

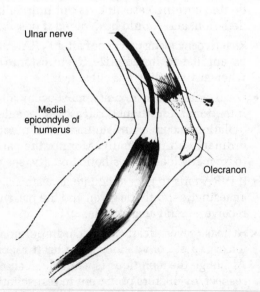

Fig. 16.4 • Ulnar nerve block at the elbow.

Landmark

The ulnar nerve can be palpated in a groove behind the medial epicondyle of the humerus.

Positioning

The patient should be supine, with the arm resting comfortably above the head and the elbow flexed at 90°

Dosage

A dose of 2–5 ml 1 per cent plain lignocaine.

Equipment

A 23 gauge × 1.25 inch (0.6 × 30 mm) needle and a 5 ml syringe.

Technique

The nerve should be blocked proximal to the ulnar groove, to reduce the risk of neuritis. Palpate the nerve in the ulnar groove, introduce the needle 1–2 cm proximally to a depth of 1–2 cm, and inject the local anaesthetic.

Onset and duration

Onset: 5–15 minutes.
Duration: 2–3 hours.

Comment

• Great care must be taken to avoid intraneural injection

Median nerve block at the elbow (Fig. 16.5)

Indications

Minor surgery in the area of innervation of the median nerve and to supplement inadequate brachial plexus block.

Special contraindications

None.

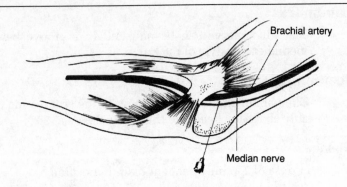

Fig. 16.5 • Median nerve block at the elbow.

Anatomy

The median nerve arises from the C5, C6, C7, C8, and T1 nerve roots, and is formed from branches of the medial and lateral cords of the brachial plexus, which unite anterior to the axillary artery. It runs lateral to the brachial artery until it reaches the mid-humerus, where it crosses to the medial side of the artery. It enters the antecubital fossa medial to the brachial artery, between the two heads of pronator teres, and is covered by the bicipital aponeurosis. It continues in the flexor compartment of the forearm.

Landmarks

The medial and lateral epicondyles and brachial artery.

Positioning

The patient should be supine, with the arm supinated comfortably at the side.

Dosage

A dose of 5 ml 1 per cent plain lignocaine.

Equipment

A 23 gauge × 1.25 inch (0.6 × 30 mm) needle and a 5 ml or 10 ml syringe.

Technique

Draw a line across the antecubital fossa between the two epicondyles. Palpate the brachial artery where it crosses the line. Insert the needle 0.5–1.0 cm medial to the brachial artery to a depth of 5 mm in a perpendicular plane. Paraesthesia may confirm that the needle has touched the nerve; withdraw 2–3 mm, and inject the local anaesthetic.

Onset and duration

Onset: 5–15 minutes.
Duration: 2–3 hours.

Comment

• Great care must be taken to avoid intraneural injection

Radial nerve and lateral cutaneous nerve of the forearm block at the elbow (Fig. 16.6)

Indications

Minor surgery in the area of innervation of the radial nerve and lateral cutaneous nerve of the forearm, and to supplement inadequate brachial plexus block.

Special contraindications

None.

Anatomy

The radial nerve arises from the C5, C6, C7, C8, and T1 nerve roots, and is the main branch of the posterior cord of the brachial plexus. It runs behind the axillary artery and passes backwards between the long and medial heads of triceps to lie in the spiral groove on the back of the humerus between the medial and lateral heads of triceps. At the level of the lower third of the humerus it pierces the lateral intermuscular septum to re-enter the anterior compartment of the arm between brachialis and brachioradialis.

The musculocutaneous nerve is derived from C5, C6, and C7, and is formed from the lateral cord of the brachial

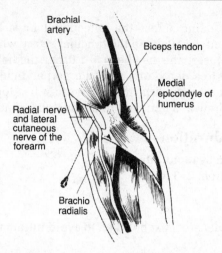

Fig. 16.6 • Radial nerve and lateral cutaneous nerve of the forearm block at the elbow.

plexus. It lies lateral to the axillary artery and pierces coracobrachialis to continue between biceps and brachialis. It forms the lateral cutaneous nerve of the forearm, which perforates the deep fascia on the lateral side of biceps just proximal to the elbow, and innervates the skin of the lateral forearm as far as the thenar eminence.

Landmarks

Medial epicondyle of the humerus, brachioradialis muscle, and biceps tendon.

Positioning

The patient should be supine, with the arm supinated comfortably at the side.

Dosage

A dose of 10–15 ml 1 per cent plain lignocaine.

Equipment

A 23 gauge × 1.25 inch (0.6 × 30 mm) needle and a 20 ml syringe.

Technique

1. To block the radial and lateral cutaneous nerve of the forearm insert the needle between the brachioradialis muscle and the biceps tendon at the level of the elbow joint.

2. Direct the needle in a proximal and lateral direction towards the lateral epicondyle of the humerus until contact is made with bone; withdraw the needle 2–3 mm and inject 2–4 ml of local anaesthetic.

3. Redirect the needle in a more cranial direction and advance it 1–3 cm in parallel with the long axis of the humerus.

4. Inject 5 ml of local anaesthetic.

If subcutaneous infiltration of local anaesthetic from the biceps to the proximal part of brachioradialis is performed the superficial branches of the musculocutaneous nerve will be blocked.

Onset and duration

Onset: 10–15 minutes.
Duration: 2–3 hours.

Comment

• Great care must be taken to avoid intraneural injection

Ulnar nerve block at the wrist (Fig. 16.7)

Indications

• Minor surgery to areas of the hand innervated by the ulnar nerve (see Fig. 16.1)
• Closed manipulation of fractures to the little finger or fifth metacarpal

Special contraindications

None.

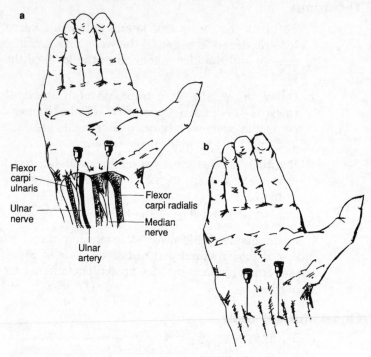

Fig. 16.7 • Ulnar and median nerve blocks at the wrist.

Anatomy

About 5 cm proximal to the wrist the ulnar nerve divides into a palmar and a dorsal cutaneous branch. The latter passes under flexor carpi ulnaris to supply the dorsum of the hand. The palmar branch lies between the ulnar artery, on its radial aspect, and flexor carpi ulnaris.

Landmarks

- The ulnar styloid process
- The ulnar artery
- Flexor carpi ulnaris

Positioning

The patient lies supine with the hand supinated and slightly flexed at the wrist.

Dosage

Palmar branch
With paraesthesia: 3–5 ml of 1 per cent lignocaine with or without adrenaline.
Without paraesthesia: 5–10 ml of 1 per cent lignocaine with or without adrenaline.

Dorsal branch
5 ml lignocaine with or without adrenaline.

Equipment

A 23 gauge × 1.25 inch (0.6 × 30 mm) needle and a 5 ml or 10 ml syringe.

Technique

Palmar branch
Introduce the needle at right angles to the skin, at the level of the ulnar styloid, between the ulnar artery and flexor carpi ulnaris. The ulnar nerve lies at a depth of 1–2 cm below the skin. If paraesthesia is elicited withdraw the needle slightly, and, after careful aspiration, inject 3–5 ml of 1 per cent lignocaine with or without adrenaline. If there is no paraesthesia insert the needle to the deep fascia and inject 5–10 ml of local anaesthetic whilst withdrawing the needle to the skin.

Dorsal branch
This is blocked by subcutaneous infiltration at the level of the ulnar styloid. Inject 5 ml 1 per cent lignocaine from flexor carpi ulnaris around the ulnar aspect of the wrist.

Onset and duration

Palmar branch
Onset: 5–10 minutes.
Duration: up to 1.5 hours.

Dorsal branch
Onset: 2–3 minutes.
Duration: up to 45 minutes.

Comments

- Before injecting local anaesthetic palpate the radial artery to confirm the presence of a collateral arterial supply to the hand. If there is any doubt adrenaline should not be used to block the palmar branch.

- A vasoconstrictor should not be used when blocking the palmar branch if there is a history of peripheral vascular disease.

- The close proximity of the ulnar artery makes careful aspiration mandatory before each injection.

- The dorsal block has a much shorter onset and duration than the palmar block, and should thus only be performed once the palmar block is established.

Median nerve block at the wrist (Fig. 16.7)

Indications

Minor surgery to areas supplied by the median nerve (Fig. 16.7).

Special contraindications

History of carpal tunnel syndrome.

Anatomy

At the level of the proximal skin crease of the wrist the median nerve lies superficially on the ulnar side of flexor carpi radialis. It may be just below or radial to the tendon of palmaris longus.

Landmarks

- Proximal skin crease of the wrist
- The tendons of palmaris longus and flexor carpi radialis

Positioning

Patient in supine position with hand supine resting comfortably at side. Clenching the fist or slight palmar flexion at the wrist may aid identification of the tendons.

Dosage

A dose of 3–5 ml 1 per cent lignocaine with or without adrenaline.

Equipment

A 23 gauge × 1.25 inch (0.6 × 30 mm) needle and a 5 ml syringe.

Technique

Insert the needle vertically between the tendons of palmaris longus and flexor carpi radialis at the level of the proximal skin crease of the wrist. At a depth of 0.5–1 cm inject 3–5 ml of 1 per cent lignocaine with or without adrenaline in a fan-shaped pattern. If paraesthesia occurs withdraw the needle slightly before injecting.

Onset and duration

Onset: 5–10 minutes.
Duration: up to 1.5 hours.

Comment

• This block may usefully be used in combination with other nerve blocks at the wrist

---

Radial nerve block at the wrist (Fig. 16.8)

Indications

Minor surgery to areas of the hand innervated by the radial nerve (Fig. 16.1).

Special contraindications

None.

Anatomy

The superficial branch is purely sensory. It lies medial to brachioradialis and at about 8 cm proximal to the wrist passes under this muscle to reach the extensor aspect of the

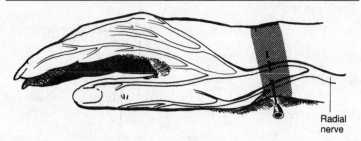

Radial
nerve

Fig. 16.8 • Radial nerve block at the wrist.

forearm. The nerve supplies a variable portion of the dorsum of the hand.

Landmark

The radial styloid.

Positioning

The patient lies supine, with the hand pronated.

Dosage

A dose of 5 ml of 0.5 per cent or 1 per cent lignocaine with or without adrenaline.

Equipment

A 23 gauge × 1.25 inch (0.6 × 30 mm) needle and a 5 ml syringe.

Technique

At the level of the radial styloid 5 ml of local anaesthetic is injected subcutaneously around the dorso-radial aspect of the wrist.

Onset and duration

Onset: 2–3 minutes.
Duration: up to 45 minutes.

Comments

- The dorso-radial aspect of the wrist has a prominent venous network. Care must be taken to avoid venepuncture or intravenous injection.

- Never infiltrate subcutaneously around the whole of the wrist, since mechanical occlusion could cause venous stasis.
- The radial nerve block at the wrist uses an infiltration technique. It therefore has a more rapid onset and shorter duration of action than the medial and ulnar blocks. The use of adrenaline prolongs the duration of the radial block, which is advantageous, particularly when used in combination with median or ulnar nerve blocks.

Combined nerve blocks at the wrist

These can be used to good effect where the operative field is supplied by more than one nerve. The radial nerve block has a much shorter onset and duration of action than the median or ulnar nerve blocks, and when used in combination should only be performed once these are established.

Digital nerve block at the metacarpal level (Fig. 16.9)

Indications

- Analgesia for injured fingers
- Simple operations on fingers

Special contraindications

None.

Anatomy

The digital nerves are formed from the median and ulnar nerves in the proximal palm. They pass distally between the flexor tendons lying on the lumbrical muscles. They lie about 0.5 cm deep to the distal palmar crease.

Landmarks

- Distal palmar crease for the fingers
- Neck of first metacarpal for the thumb

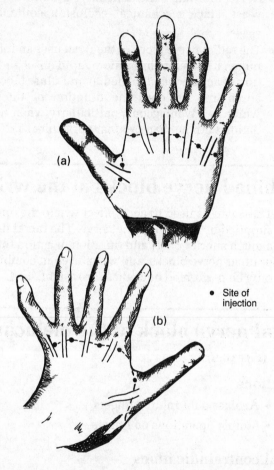

(a)

• Site of injection

(b)

Fig. 16.9 • Digital nerve block at the metacarpal level: (a) palmar view; (b) dorsal view.

Positioning

The patient is supine with the forearm supinated and the hand resting comfortably.

Dosage

A dose of 5 ml of 1 per cent plain lignocaine.

Equipment

A 23 gauge × 1.25 inch (0.6 × 30 mm) needle or a 25 gauge × 0.6 inch (0.5 × 16 mm) needle for small children and a 2 or 5 ml syringe.

Technique

Identify the appropriate nerves to be blocked. With a palmar approach inject 1.5–2.0 ml of 1 per cent plain lignocaine :about 0.5 cm deep to the skin at the level of the palmar crease. A further dose of 1–2 ml of plain lignocaine may be infiltrated over the dorsum of the metacarpal spaces to block small dorsal nerves.

Onset and duration

Onset: 2–5 minutes.
Duration: 45 minutes to 1 hour.

Comments

- Never use a vasoconstrictor.
- A block at this level usually affects the digital nerve to the adjacent finger. This is of value when more than one finger requires treatment.
- A dorsal approach may be used for this technique, but carries an increased risk of venepuncture. The digital nerves also lie further from the dorsal skin and may be more difficult to block. The dorsal approach is claimed to be less painful; but if a fine needle is used through the palmar crease discomfort is minimal.

Digital nerve block at the base of the digit

(Fig. 16.10)

Indications

Simple operations on the distal two-thirds of fingers or toes.

Special contraindications

None.

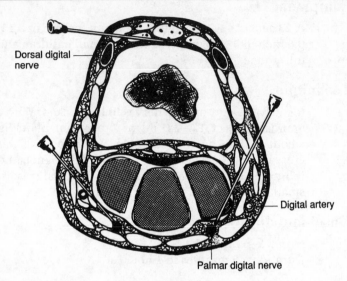

Fig. 16.10 • Digital nerve block at the base of the digit.

Anatomy

A dorsal and palmar (plantar) nerve run along each side of the digit.

Landmark

Base of the digit dorsally.

Positioning

Patient in supine position with limb resting comfortably.

Dosage

A dose of 2–5 ml of 1 per cent plain lignocaine.

Equipment

A 23 gauge × 1.25 inch (0.6 × 30 mm) needle or a 25 gauge × 0.6 inch (0.5 × 16 mm) needle for small children and a 2 or 5 ml syringe.

Technique

1. Using a dorsal approach, introduce the needle at the base

of the radial side of the digit until the needle can be felt on the flexor surface.

2. Inject 0.5–1.5 ml of plain lignocaine while slowly withdrawing the needle.
3. Repeat on the ulnar aspect.
4. Inject 0.5–1.5 ml across the dorsum of the digit.

Onset and duration

Onset: 2–5 minutes.
Duration: 45 minutes to 1 hour.

Comments

- Never use a vasoconstrictor.
- This technique is often called a `ring block', implying that local anaesthetic is put all around the finger like a ring. This should be avoided, since it increases the risk of ischaemia caused by the mass of local anaesthetic producing vascular occlusion.
- The maximum volume of local anaesthetic used at the base of a digit is 5 ml. This should be reduced in smaller digits, such as toes, or in children.

Infiltration of fracture haematoma

Indications

- Not for routine use
- Reduction of wrist fractures in a mass casualty situation

Special contraindications

- Fractures over 24 hours old
- Infection of the skin overlying the fracture

Anatomy

Nerves supplying the periosteum, bone, and surrounding soft tissue are blocked by direct local infiltration.

Landmark

Fracture site.

Positioning

The patient lies supine, with the arm resting comfortably at the side.

Dosage

A dose of 15 ml of 1 per cent plain prilocaine or lignocaine.

Equipment

A 23 gauge × 1.25 inch (0.6 × 30 mm) needle and a 20 ml syringe.

Technique

Use aseptic technique. Insert the needle into the haematoma and confirm its position by positive aspiration. The local anaesthetic should be injected very slowly, to reduce the risk of delivering a bolus dose into the circulation, and to minimize pain. Anaesthesia of the distal radial ulna joint may also be needed when using this technique.

Onset and duration

Onset: 5 minutes.
Duration: up to 1 hour.

Comments

- **Never** use a vasoconstrictor, as rapid absorption may cause toxicity.
- The technique converts a closed into an open fracture; thus a careful aseptic technique is required.
- Rapid absorption of local anaesthetic from the haematoma or from inadvertent intravascular injection may cause toxicity. It is difficult to tell on aspiration whether blood is coming from the haematoma or from a punctured vessel; therefore always be alert to the signs of toxicity.
- Analgesia by this method is sometimes barely adequate.
- This technique should not be used if the fracture is over 24 hours old, since haematoma organization will prevent the spread of local anaesthetic.

Further reading

Casualty Surgeons' Association (1983). *Bier's blocks (intravenous regional anaesthesia): code of practice.* The Association, London.

Cobb, A. G. and Houghton, G. R. (1985). Local anaesthetic infiltration versus Bier's block for Colles' fractures. *British Medical Journal*, **291**, 1683–4.

Goldberg, M. E., Gregg, C., Larijani, G. E., Norris, M. C., Marr, A. T., and Seltzer, J. L. (1987). A comparison of three methods of axillary approach to brachial plexus blockade for upper extremity surgery. *Anesthesiology*, **66**, 814–16.

Goold, J. E. (1985). Intravenous regional anaesthesia. *British Journal of Hospital Medicine*, **33**, 335–40.

Henderson, A. M. (1980). Adverse reactions to bupivacaine—complications of intravenous regional anaesthesia. *British Medical Journal*, **281**, 1043–4.

Partridge, B. L., Katz, J., and Benirschke, K. (1987). Functional anatomy of the brachial plexus sheath: implications for anesthesia. *Anesthesiology*, **66**, 743–7.

Selander, D. (1987). Axillary plexus block: paresthetic or perivascular. *Anesthesiology*, **66**, 726–8.

Tucker, G. T. and Boas, R. A. (1971). Pharmacokinetic aspects of intravenous regional anaesthesia. *Anesthesiology*, **34**, 538–49.

Wallace, W. A., Guardini, R., and Ellis, S. J. (1982). Standard intravenous regional anaesthesia. *British Medical Journal*, **285**, 554–6.

Winnie, A. P. (1970). Interscalene brachial plexus block. *Anesthesia and Analgesia*, **49**, 455–65.

Winnie, A. P. (1984). *Plexus anaesthsia*, Vol. 1. Churchill Livingstone, Edinburgh.

Winnie, A. P. and Collins, V. J. (1964). The subclavian perivascular technique of brachial plexus anesthesia. *Anesthesiology*, **25**, 353–63.

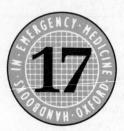

CHAPTER 17

Nerve blocks of the lower limb

Sciatic nerve block

Indications

Anaesthesia and analgesia of the lower limb if combined with a femoral or 3 in 1 block (see p. 343). The pain of hip, tibial, or femoral shaft fracture may be treated by combined sciatic and femoral nerve blocks. Posterior and anterior approaches to the sciatic nerve are described. In the A & E setting, when the block is used during the management of trauma, the anterior approach is preferable, as it can be performed with the patient supine. The posterior approach requires that the patient is turned laterally.

Special contraindications

None.

Anatomy

The sciatic nerve arises from the sacral plexus and has contributions from the L4, L5, S1, S2, and S3 nerve roots. It leaves the pelvis, with the posterior cutaneous nerve of the thigh and the inferior gluteal artery, via the greater sciatic notch. It is covered by gluteus maximus and runs down the surface of gemelli, obturator internus, and quadratus femoris to pass a point which lies equidistant from the posterior superior ischial spine and the greater trochanter. It continues in the posterior compartment of the thigh. It lies immediately posterior to the lesser trochanter and is covered anteriorly by iliopsoas, rectus femoris, and sartorius. The

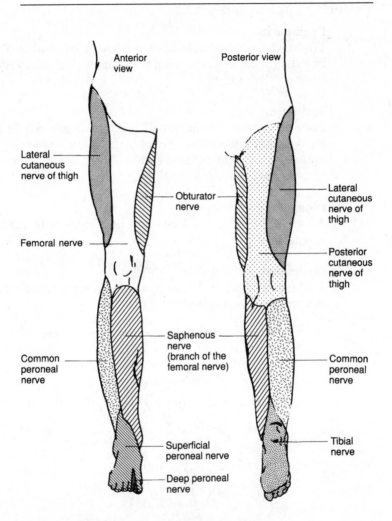

Fig. 17.1 • Cutaneous innervation of the lower limb.

sciatic nerve divides above the popliteal fossa to form the common peroneal and tibial nerves, which supply the foot and the postero-lateral aspect of the calf. The posterior aspect of the thigh is supplied by the posterior cutaneous nerve of the thigh. Figure 17.1 shows a simplified diagram of the innervation of the lower limb.

Posterior approach (Fig. 17.2)

Landmarks
The sciatic nerve crosses 3–4 cm below the midpoint of a line drawn between the greater trochanter and the posterior superior iliac spine.

Positioning
Place the patient in the lateral position with the side to be blocked uppermost. The lower leg should be straight and the upper leg flexed at 45° and adducted so that the upper knee rests on the bed anterior to the lower leg.

Dosage
A dose of 20–30 ml of 1 per cent lignocaine with 1:200 000 adrenaline.

Equipment
A 23 gauge × 3.5 inch (0.6 × 84 mm) short bevelled needle and two 20 ml syringes.

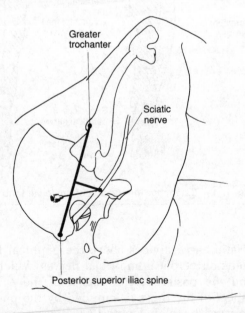

Greater trochanter

Sciatic nerve

Posterior superior iliac spine

Fig. 17.2 • Sciatic nerve block: posterior approach.

Technique

1. Mark the position of the posterior superior iliac spine and the posterior superior end of the greater trochanter and join the marks by a line; place the upper leg so that the long axis of the femur forms a continuation of the line.

2. Mark the midpoint of the line and draw a line perpendicular to the midpoint 3–4 cm long to show the site for needle insertion.

3. Insert the needle at 90° to the skin in all planes, to a depth of 6–8 cm. Paraesthesia may occur in the sciatic nerve distribution. More than one injection may give better results because of the size of the sciatic nerve. The tibial and peroneal branches can be identified separately using a PNS. 10 ml of local anaesthetic injected into each component may produce a better block. This will still block the posterior femoral cutaneous nerve.

4. After negative aspiration inject the local anaesthetic.

Onset and duration
Onset: 15–30 minutes.
Duration: 4–6 hours.

Anterior approach (Fig. 17.3)

Landmarks
The anterior approach uses a line drawn between the anterior superior iliac spine and the pubic tubercle, and a line drawn parallel to this from the greater trochanter, to locate the position of the sciatic nerve as it passes posterior to the lesser trochanter.

Positioning
The patient should be supine, with the hip abducted at 10° and externally rotated.

Dosage
20–35 ml of 1 per cent lignocaine with 1:200 000 adrenaline.

Equipment
A 23 gauge × 3.5 inch (0.6 × 84 mm) short bevelled needle and a 20 ml syringe.

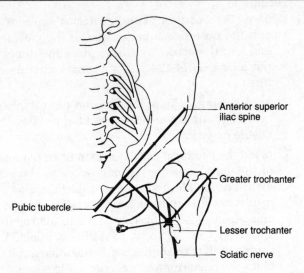

Fig. 17.3 • Sciatic nerve block: anterior approach.

Technique

1. Draw a line joining the anterior superior iliac spine and the pubic tubercle and divide this equally into three; then draw a second line parallel to this from the superior part of the greater trochanter.

2. Draw a perpendicular line caudally and laterally from a point joining the medial and middle third of the first line to impinge on the second line. The point where the perpendicular line meets the second line marks the position for needle insertion.

3. Insert the needle perpendicular to the skin, and advance it until it strikes the anterior surface of the femur, at a depth of 8–10 cm.

4. Withdraw the needle and redirect it so that it just slides off the medial surface of the femur and pierces the adductor muscles.

5. Attach a syringe filled with air or saline and advance the needle up to 5 cm further, with pressure on the barrel of the syringe; resistance to injection suddenly disappears as the needle enters the posterior compartment of the thigh.

6. After negative aspiration, inject the local anaesthetic.

Onset and duration
Onset: 15–30 minutes.
Duration: 4–6 hours.

Comments

- The success of sciatic block is improved by the use of a nerve stimulator.
- A large mass of local anaesthetic is needed to block the whole lower limb. It is important to remain within safe dose limits.
- The posterior cutaneous nerve of the thigh is often blocked during the posterior approach to the sciatic nerve.

The 3 in 1 block (Fig. 17.4)

Indications

The 3 in 1 block affects the femoral nerve, the obturator nerve, and the lateral cutaneous nerve of the thigh. It anaesthetizes the anterior, medial, and lateral aspects of the thigh. It can be used in combination with a sciatic block to anaesthetize the lower limb. However, care must be taken not to exceed the toxic dose of local anaesthetic. It may be necessary to reduce the local anaesthetic concentration (not the volume) slightly to remain within safe dose limits.

Special contraindications

None.

Anatomy

The femoral and obturator nerves arise from the lumbar plexus and have contributions from the L2, L3, and L4 nerve roots. The femoral nerve emerges from the lateral border of the psoas muscle and runs deep to the iliac fascia in a groove between psoas and iliacus. It enters the thigh beneath the inguinal ligament, lateral to the femoral artery, and is

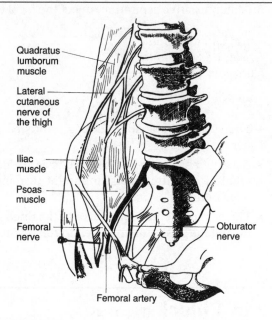

Fig. 17.4 • 3 in 1 block.

enclosed in a fascial sheath. The femoral nerve supplies the anterior thigh, the medial side of the calf and the extensors of the knee. The obturator nerve emerges from the medial border of psoas at the level of the sacroiliac joint. It crosses the sacral ala and passes along the pelvic wall via the obturator canal to enter the medial muscular compartment of the thigh. The obturator nerve supplies a small area of skin on the medial aspect of the thigh and the adductors of the hip. The lateral cutaneous nerve of the thigh arises from the lumbar plexus, with contributions from L2 and L3 nerve roots. It runs obliquely downward and forwards on the iliac muscle. It passes deep to the inguinal ligament 1–2 cm medial to the anterior superior iliac spine, to enter the thigh and supply the lateral aspect of the thigh.

Landmarks

- The inguinal ligament
- The femoral artery

Positioning

The patient is supine, with the hip slightly abducted and externally rotated.

Dosage

A dose of 25–30 ml of 1 per cent lignocaine with 1:200 000 adrenaline in an adult.

Equipment

A 23 gauge × 3.5 inch (0.6 × 84 mm) needle; an extension for remote injection; and two 20 ml syringes.

Technique

1. Palpate the femoral artery at the point where it emerges beneath the inguinal ligament.

2. Insert the needle 1.0–1.5 cm lateral to the femoral artery, guarding the artery with the index finger to prevent accidental puncture. Aim perpendicular to the skin or slightly cranially. A click may be felt as the needle pierces the fascia lata at a depth of about 1.5–3.0 cm in an adult; this is followed by a second click as the needle pierces the fascia iliaca, about 0.5 cm deeper.

3. Apply pressure distal to the point of insertion of the needle and inject 25–30 ml of local anaesthetic for an adult. Maintain the pressure for 5 minutes.

Onset and duration

Onset: 15–30 minutes.
Duration: 4–6 hours.

Comments

- The success of a 3 in 1 block can be improved by the use of a nerve stimulator.

- The site of injection is the same for femoral and 3 in 1 blocks. The larger volume of local anaesthetic used and the application of digital pressure distal to the injection site during a 3 in 1 block result in proximal spread of local anaesthetic solution up the psoas sheath, which contains the obturator and femoral nerves and the lateral cutaneous nerve of the thigh.

Femoral nerve block (Fig. 17.5)

Indications

- Analgesia for a fractured shaft of femur, including the application of traction.
- Analgesia for a fractured patella.
- Anaesthetizing the donor area for a skin graft. (Often used in combination with lateral cutaneous nerve block. See also 3 in 1 block.)

Special contraindications

None.

Anatomy

See p. 343.

Landmarks

- The inguinal ligament
- The femoral artery

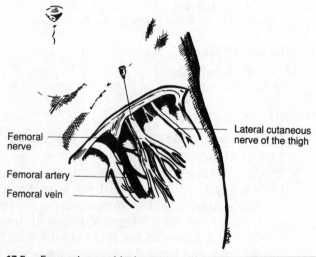

Femoral nerve

Lateral cutaneous nerve of the thigh

Femoral artery

Femoral vein

Fig. 17.5 • Femoral nerve block.

Positioning

The patient should lie supine, with the leg resting flat and slightly abducted. This position may not be possible in patients with a fractured shaft of the femur. The best position obtainable, without distressing the patient, should be accepted in this case.

Dosage

A dose of 10–15 ml of 1 per cent lignocaine with or without adrenaline.

Equipment

- A 21 gauge × 1.5 inch (0.8 × 40 mm) needle for adults
- A 23 gauge × 1.25 inch (0.6 × 30 mm) needle for children
- A 25 gauge × 0.6 inch (0.5 × 16 mm) needle for infants
- A 2, 5, 10, or 20 ml syringe, depending on the size of patient.

Technique

1. Place one finger over the femoral artery as it emerges under the inguinal ligament.
2. Insert the needle just lateral to this, perpendicular to the skin.
3. Advance the needle 1 to 4 cm.
4. If paraesthesia is elicited withdraw the needle slightly, and after careful aspiration, slowly inject 10 ml of 1 per cent lignocaine with adrenaline. Otherwise inject 10 to 15 ml of local anaesthetic whilst the needle is moved from a depth of 4 cm up and down, gradually moving 3 cm lateral from the artery. Aspirate carefully before each injection.

Onset and duration

Onset: 5–15 minutes.
Duration: up to 1.5 hours.

Comments

- This technique uses a large dose of lignocaine, care must be taken not to exceed the maximum dose. It is often impossible to know the patient's weight accurately. For children age/weight charts may be used. By using lignocaine with adrenaline the maximum safe dose is almost doubled. The duration of action is also increased.

- Bupivicaine is a useful alternative to plain lignocaine, as it has a longer duration of action. A dose of 10 ml of 0.5 per cent plain bupivicaine may be used for an adult.

- This technique is useful for providing analgesia for a fractured shaft of the femur and may be used in pre-hospital care. It is most effective for fractures of the mid-shaft, with diminishing efficacy for fractures of the distal third and finally the proximal third. Care must be taken that nerve blocking does not mask a compartment syndrome.

- This block is suitable for all ages. It has been used safely and successfully in one year olds. The importance of using the correct dose cannot be stressed too much.

- If the femoral artery is punctured, compress it for 5–10 minutes. If there is no evidence of bleeding continue with the procedure.

- This block is usually easy to perform. Problems occasionally arise when the femoral artery is difficult to palpate, as may occur in the obese or those with peripheral vascular disease. Some small children with a fractured femur hold their leg flexed at the hip, preventing adequate positioning. In this case alternative analgesia should be given. A femoral nerve block may be possible at a later stage if the leg can be repositioned without causing any distress.

- Local anaesthetic with adrenaline should be avoided in patients with peripheral vascular disease.

Intravenous regional anaesthesia (IVRA) of the lower limb

Indications

IVRA can be used to provide anaesthesia for surgery or fracture manipulation for one leg below the knee. IVRA is less commonly used in the lower limb than in the upper limb, because of problems with the application of a tourniquet and the larger dose of local anaesthetic needed for the leg.

Special contraindica]tions

As for the upper limb (see p. 315). Also a history of a deep-vein thrombosis in the lower limb contraindicates IVRA.

Anatomy and positioning

As for the upper limb (see p. 315).

Dosage

A dose of 40–60 ml of 0.5 per cent prilocaine is needed to anaesthetize the lower limb. If this exceeds the toxic dose for an individual IVRA is contraindicated.

Equipment

As for the upper limb (see p. 315), with a wider tourniquet.

Technique

IVRA in the lower limb is performed in the same way as for the upper limb (see p. 315) apart from the tourniquet placement and the dose of prilocaine. The cuff can be placed either above the knee, which increases the volume of prilocaine required because of the larger mass of isolated limb, or below the knee, with a risk of compression of the peroneal nerve or deep vein thrombosis. The tourniquet should be inflated to 400 mmHg.

Onset and duration

As for the upper limb (see p. 315).

Comments

Fagg (1987) described 50 patients having IVRA for surgery on the lower limb. The tourniquet was applied below the neck of the fibula, where the common peroneal nerve is well protected by muscle, and 40 ml of 0.5 per cent prilocaine were used. There were 10 cases of tourniquet failure (two accidental and eight during inflation of a double cuff); four patients needed intravenous diazepam for 'agitation'; two patients experienced severe tourniquet pain; and 1 patient had a deep-vein thrombosis. When a calf tourniquet is used the leakage into the systemic circulation is twice that of an arm tourniquet. It does not depend on height, weight, limb volume, or limb circumference. As alternative methods for anaesthesia for the lower limb are available, they should usually be chosen in preference to IVRA.

Tibial nerve block (Fig. 17.6)

Indications

Minor operations to the sole of the foot (usually in combination with a sural nerve block).

Special contraindications

None.

Anatomy

The tibial nerve lies medial to the Achilles tendon. It passes behind the posterior tibial artery and between the tendons of flexor digitorum longus and flexor hallucis longus under

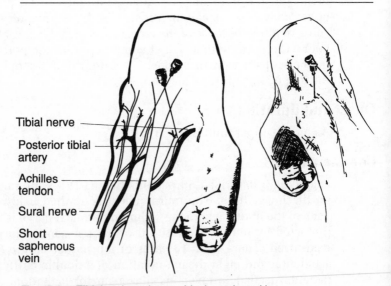

Fig. 17.6 • Tibial and sural nerve blocks at the ankle.

cover of the flexor retinaculum. At the back of the medial malleolus it divides into the medial and lateral plantar nerves, which supply the sole of the foot. A small branch supplies the medial aspect of the heel (Fig. 17.7).

Landmarks

- Medial malleolus
- Achilles tendon
- Posterior tibial artery

Positioning

The patient lies prone, with the legs extended. The ankle is supported by a pillow and the foot is slightly dorsiflexed.

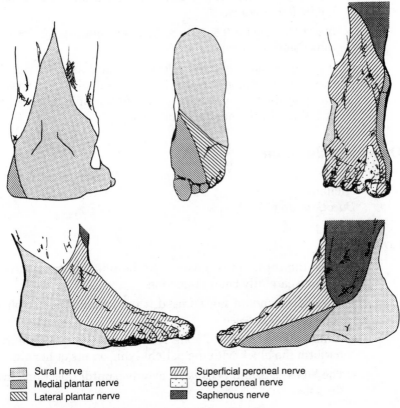

▨ Sural nerve		⧄ Superficial peroneal nerve	
▨ Medial plantar nerve		⋰ Deep peroneal nerve	
▨ Lateral plantar nerve		▨ Saphenous nerve	

Fig. 17.7 • Cutaneous innervation of the foot and ankle.

Dosage

A dose of 5–10 ml of 1 per cent lignocaine with or without adrenaline.

Equipment

A 23 gauge × 1.25 inch (0.6 × 30 mm) or 25 gauge × 0.6 inch (0.5 × 16 mm) needle and a 10 ml syringe.

Technique

1. Palpate the tibial artery.
2. Insert the needle vertically and slightly lateral to the posterior tibial artery. If the artery cannot be felt, insert the needle next to the Achilles tendon at the level of the medical malleolus.
3. Insert the needle 0.5–2.0 cm deep and perpendicular to the posterior aspect of the tibia.
4. If paraesthesia is elicited inject 5 ml local anaesthetic. If there are no paraesthesiae, inject 10 ml of local anaesthetic against the posterior aspect of the tibia, gradually withdrawing the needle about 1 cm.

Onset and duration

Onset: 5–10 minutes (up to 30 minutes if paraesthesia is not elicited).
Duration: up to 1.5 hours.

Comments

- Since the injection is adjacent to the tibial artery always aspirate carefully before injection
- Adrenaline should not be used if the patient has peripheral vascular disease
- If the patient cannot tolerate lying prone it is possible to perform the block with the patient lying on his or her side
- The block is useful because it avoids painful injections in the sole

Sural nerve block (Fig. 17.6)

Indications

Minor operations to the sole of the foot (usually in combination with a tibial nerve block).

Special contraindications

None.

Anatomy

The sural nerve passes behind the lateral malleolus, with the saphenous vein, to supply the lateral margin of the foot.

Landmarks

- Lateral malleolus
- Achilles tendon

Positioning

The patient lies prone, with the legs extended. The ankle rests on a pillow, with the foot slightly dorsiflexed.

Dosage

A dose of 5–8 ml of 0.5 or 1 per cent lignocaine with adrenaline.

Equipment

A 23 gauge × 1.25 inch (0.6 × 30 mm) or 25 gauge × 0.6 inch (0.5 × 16 mm) needle and a 10 ml syringe.

Technique

Infiltrate the subcutaneous tissue between the Achilles tendon and the lateral malleolus with 5 to 8 ml of 1 per cent lignocaine with adrenaline.

Onset and duration

Onset: 2–3 minutes.
Duration: up to 1 hour.

Comments

- Care should be taken to avoid puncture of the prominent venous system at this site.
- This block has a shorter onset and duration than a tibial nerve block. When used with the latter it should not be started until the tibial nerve block is established.

Superficial peroneal nerve block (Fig. 17.8)

Indications

Minor operations to the foot (usually in combination with other nerve blocks at the ankle).

Special contraindications

None.

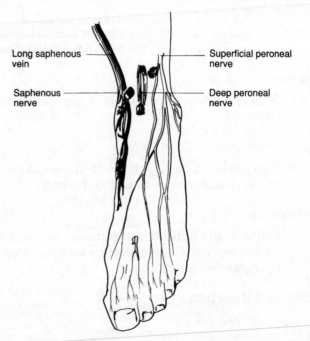

Long saphenous vein

Saphenous nerve

Superficial peroneal nerve

Deep peroneal nerve

Fig. 17.8 • Anterior ankle blocks.

Anatomy

The superficial peroneal nerve perforates the crural fascia in the distal two-thirds of the lower leg. It passes subcutaneously to supply the dorsum of the foot and toes (Fig. 17.7).

Landmarks

- Anterior border of tibia
- Lateral malleolus

Positioning

The patient lies supine, with the leg extended and the foot slightly plantar-flexed.

Dosage

A dose of 5–10 ml of 0.5 or 1 per cent lignocaine with adrenaline.

Equipment

A 23 gauge × 1.25 inch (0.6 × 30 mm) or 25 gauge × 0.6 inch (0.5 × 16 mm) needle and a 10 ml syringe.

Technique

Infiltrate 5 – 10 ml local anaesthetic subcutaneously between the lateral malleolus and the anterior border of the tibia.

Onset and duration

Onset: 2–3 minutes.
Duration: up to 1 hour.

Combined sural and superficial peroneal nerve block

Indications

Minor operations to the foot.

Special contraindications

None.

Anatomy

See p. 353.

Landmarks

- Lateral malleolus
- Anterior tibial edge
- Achilles tendon

Positioning

The patient lies on his or her side, with the leg to be anaesthetized uppermost. However, the patient may also lie prone or supine, depending on what other blocks are to be performed.

Dosage

A dose of 10–20 ml of 0.5 per cent lignocaine with adrenaline.

Equipment

A 23 gauge × 1.25 inch (0.6 × 30 mm) or 25 gauge × 0.6 inch (0.5 × 16 mm) needle and a 10 or 20 ml syringe.

Technique

About one hand's breadth proximal to the lateral malleolus infiltrate the local anaesthetic subcutaneously in a line parallel to the upper ankle joint from the anterior tibial edge laterally around to the Achilles tendon.

Onset and duration

Onset: 2–3 minutes.
Duration: up to 1 hour.

Deep peroneal nerve block (Fig. 17.8)

Indications

Minor operations to the foot (in combination with other nerve blocks at the ankle).

Special contraindications

None.

Anatomy

The deep peroneal nerve passes under the extensor retinaculum of the ankle with the dorsalis pedis artery. It continues between the tendons of extensor hallucis longus and extensor digitorum communis. The nerve lies laterally or inferiorly to the dorsalis pedis artery and continues distally to innervate the skin between the first and second toes (Fig. 17.7).

Landmarks

- Dorsalis pedis artery
- Extensor hallucis longus tendon

Positioning

The patient lies supine, with the leg extended and the foot plantar-flexed.

Dosage

A dose of 4–6 ml of 1 per cent lignocaine with or without adrenaline.

Equipment

A 23 gauge × 1.25 inch (0.6 × 30 mm) or 25 gauge × 0.6 inch (0.5 × 16 mm) needle and a 10 ml syringe.

Technique

1. Locate the dorsalis pedis artery and introduce the needle immediately medial to it at right angles to the skin.
2. With the needle tip directly next to or slightly below the artery inject 2 to 3 ml of local anaesthetic.
3. In view of anatomic variations, repeat this procedure on the lateral side of the artery.

Onset and duration

Onset: 5–10 minutes.
Duration: up to 1 hour.

Comments

- Close proximity of the artery requires that careful negative aspiration should always be obtained before injecting local anaesthetic
- Adrenaline should not be used if there is a history of peripheral vascular disease

---

Saphenous nerve block (Fig. 17.8)

Indications

Minor operations to the foot (in combination with other nerve blocks at the ankle).

Special contraindications

None.

Anatomy

The saphenous nerve passes distally with the great saphenous vein and reaches the medial surface of the ankle between the medial malleolus and the edge of the tibia. It provides the sensory innervation to the medial malleolus and the medial aspect of the foot (Fig. 17.7).

Landmarks

- Anterior tibial edge
- Medial malleolus
- Achilles tendon

Positioning

The patient lies supine, with the leg slightly externally rotated at the hip and flexed at the knee. The patient may lie prone if necessary.

Dosage

A dose of 5–10 ml of 0.5 or 1 per cent lignocaine with or without adrenaline.

Equipment

A 23 gauge × 1.25 inch (0.6 × 30 mm) or 25 gauge × 0.6 inch (0.5 × 16 mm) needle and a 10 ml syringe.

Technique

Approximately one hand's breadth proximal to the medial malleolus inject the local anaesthetic subcutaneously from the anterior tibial edge medially around to the Achilles tendon.

Onset and duration

Onset: within 2 minutes.
Duration: up to 1 hour.

Compartment block to the lower limb

Indications

To block the tibial and common peroneal nerves for surgery to the foot.

Special contraindications

Care must be taken not to mask a compartment syndrome with this block.

Anatomy

The lower leg may be divided into anterior, peroneal, and posterior compartments. Each contains a group of similarly functioning muscles and a neurvascular bundle. The nerves run in an enclosed space surrounded by fascial sheaths. If local anaesthetic is injected into a compartment it will reach the appropriate nerves. This technique decreases the risk of neurovascular trauma. The anterior compartment is anterior to the tibia, fibula, and interosseous membrane. Its lateral boundary is the anterior crural or peroneal fascial septum. It contains the extensors and inverters of the foot and the deep peroneal nerve. The peroneal compartment is bordered by the fibula, with its attached anterior and posterior crural membrane or peroneal septa, and the deep fascia of the leg. It contains the everters of the foot and the superior peroneal nerve. The common peroneal nerve enters this compartment before dividing. The posterior compartment is bounded anteriorly by the tibia, fibula, and interosseous membrane. It is subdivided by a posterior septum into a superficial subcompartment containing the foot flexors and a deep subcompartment containing the toe flexors and the tibial nerve.

Posterior compartment block (tibial nerve)

Landmarks
The tibial nerve lies under the cover of the posterior intramuscular septum. It runs inferior and in direct relationship to the toe flexors.

Positioning
Place the patient supine.

Dosage
10–15 ml of 1 per cent lignocaine with or without adrenaline.

Equipment
Peripheral nerve stimulator and 3.5 inch (84 mm) insulated needle.

Technique
1. Approach the compartment medially with the needle aimed directly at the deep posterior compartment. Introduce the needle perpendicular to the medial surface of the tibia just posterior to the medial border of the tibia at the level of the tibial tubercle. The needle depth should be nearly equal to the medial subcutaneous surface of the fibula.
2. Locate the tibial nerve with a PNS to produce toe flexion.
3. Inject 10–15 ml of local anaesthetic.

Peroneal compartment block (common peroneal nerve)

Landmark
The common peroneal nerve is blocked in the compartment before it divides.

Positioning
Place the patient supine.

Dosage
5–10 ml of 1 per cent lignocaine with or without adrenaline.

Equipment
2.5 inch (60 mm) needle.

Technique
1. Palpate the head of the fibula at the insertion of biceps femoris. Place the needle 2.5 cm inferior to the head of the fibula in a horizontal direction. Aim at the lateral surface of the fibula, not at the nerve, until bone is contacted.
2. Withdraw the needle 1–2 mm and inject 5–10 ml of local anaesthetic.

Onset and duration

Onset: the block is complete within 45 minutes.
Duration: 4–6 hours.

Comment

- The compartment block may be supplemented by infiltration of the saphenous nerve (see p. 358).

Combined nerve blocks at the ankle

The foot is innervated by five terminal branches from the lumbosacral plexus, namely the tibial, sural, saphenous, deep peroneal, and superficial peroneal nerves. These have a variable cutaneous distribution and it is therefore wise to use combined nerve blocks. Care must always be taken when using these blocks to ensure that the maximum total dose of local anaesthetic is not exceeded. Using adrenaline for the subcutaneous infiltration techniques will not only give a wider margin of safety, but will also prolong the duration of block. Never inject a complete ring of local anaesthetic around the leg, as this could compromise the circulation. If saphenous, sural, and superficial peroneal blocks are required they should be done at different levels.

Digital nerve block at the base of the toe

This technique is described on p. 333. Although the big toe may require 5 ml of local anaesthetic, the other toes often require much smaller volumes. Never use a vasoconstrictor.

Further reading

Casualty Surgeons' Association (1983). *Bier's blocks (intravenous regional anaesthesia): code of practice.* The Association, London.

Fagg, P. S. (1987). Intravenous regional anaesthesia for lower limb orthopaedic surgery. *Annals of the Royal College of Surgeons*, **69**, 274–5.

Goold, J. E. (1985). Intravenous regional anaesthesia. *British Journal of Hospital Medicine*, **33**, 335–40.

Henderson, A. M. (1980). Adverse reactions to bupivacaine—complications of intravenous regional anaesthesia. *British Medical Journal*, **281**, 1043–4.

Tucker, G. T. and Boas, R. A. (1971). Pharmacokinetic aspects of intravenous regional anaesthesia. *Anesthesiology*, **34**, 538–49.

Wallace, W. A., Guardini, R., and Ellis, S. J. (1982). Standard intravenous regional anaesthesia. *British Medical Journal*, **285**, 554–6.

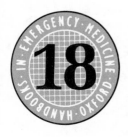

CHAPTER 18

Other nerve blocks and field blocks

Supraorbital and supratrochlear nerve block (Fig. 18.1)

Indications

Minor surgical procedures to the forehead and frontal region of the scalp.

Special contraindications

Open skull fractures in the area of the block.

Anatomy

The supraorbital nerve leaves the orbit as two branches through two holes or notches on the superior orbital margin about 2.5 cm from the midline. It supplies the skin of the forehead, including adjacent scalp. The supratrochlear nerve leaves the orbit medial to the supraorbital nerve. It provides cutaneous sensation to the medial part of the forehead.

Landmarks

- The root of the nose
- The upper margin of the eyebrow

Positioning

The patient lies supine, with the head resting comfortably.

Dosage

A dose of 5–10 ml of 1 per cent lignocaine with or without adrenaline.

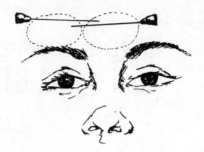

Fig. 18.1 • Supraorbital and supratrochlear nerve block.

Equipment

A 23 gauge × 1.25 inch (0.6 × 30 mm) or 25 gauge × 0.6 inch (0.5 × 16 mm) needle and a 5 or 10 ml syringe.

Technique

1. Insert the needle in the midline between the eyebrows and direct it laterally.
2. Inject 5 to 10 ml of local anaesthetic from the point of entry along the upper margin of the eyebrow.

Onset and duration

Onset: 2–3 minutes.
Duration: up to 1 hour.

Comments

- The lateral extremes of the forehead may be outside the field of the block. In this case the needle should be reinserted within the lateral limit of the first injection, and the block should be extended laterally by further local infiltration.
- Needle injury to the eye may occur if the patient is uncooperative or the operator is careless.
- Inadvertent orbital injection may cause temporary blindness if the optic nerve is involved.

Field block of the ear

Indications

Lacerations of the pinna.

Special contraindications

None.

Anatomy

The pinna is supplied by sensory branches of the greater occipital, lesser occipital, and auriculotemporal nerves. These travel subcutaneously to the ear.

Landmarks

- Base of the ear lobe
- Temporal artery

Positioning

The patient lies supine. The head is turned with the operative side uppermost and supported on a pillow or head-ring.

Dosage

A dose of 10–15 ml of 0.5 or 1 per cent plain lignocaine.

Equipment

A 23 gauge × 1.25 inch (0.6 × 30 mm) or 25 gauge × 0.6 inch (0.5 × 16 mm) needle and a 10 or 20 ml syringe.

Technique

1. Insert the needle 1 cm below the base of the ear lobe.
2. Direct the needle anterior and posterior to the ear, injecting local anaesthetic subcutaneously.
3. Reinsert the needle into the anaesthetized areas and complete the subcutaneous injection of a ring of local anaesthetic around the ear.

Onset and duration

Onset: 2–3 minutes.
Duration: up to 45 minutes.

Comments

- The pinna is supplied by end-arteries; thus a vasoconstrictor should *never* be used
- Always aspirate carefully to avoid an intravascular injection into the temporal artery

Stellate ganglion block (Fig. 18.2)

Indications

- The sympathetic nerve supply to the head, neck, and arm can be interrupted at the stellate ganglion to produce vasodilatation
- Vascular insufficiency and pain
- Treatment of accidental intra-arterial injection of irritant solutions, such as thiopentone

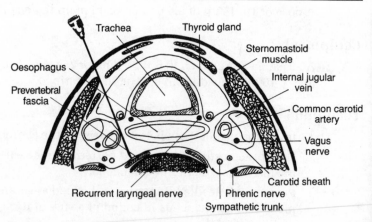

Fig. 18.2 • Stellate ganglion block.

Special contraindications

- There is potential for adverse effects after stellate ganglion block so it should be used with caution in patients with severe cardiorespiratory problems
- Simultaneous bilateral blocks should be avoided, as bilateral phrenic or recurrent laryngeal nerve block may occur

Anatomy

The stellate ganglion is formed by fusion of the inferior cervical ganglion with the upper thoracic ganglion. The sympathetic chain travels upwards from the thorax, crosses the neck of the first rib, and ascends to the skull base, embedded in the posterior wall of the carotid sheath. The sympathetic chain lies anterior to the fascia covering the prevertebral muscles, which form a thin layer over the transverse processes of the cervical vertebrae. The transverse process of the sixth cervical vertebra can be palpated at the level of the cricoid cartilage. The vertebral artery runs upwards enclosed in foramina in the transverse processes, and the cervical spinal nerves pass out between the transverse processes encased in long dural sleeves. The carotid sheath lies anterior to the sympathetic chain; the pharynx, oesophagus, and larynx lie medially; and the recurrent laryngeal nerve runs between them. The dome of the pleura lies inferior to the stellate ganglion.

Landmarks

The transverse process of C6 is palpated at, or slightly above, the level of the cricoid cartilage and carotid pulsation is felt laterally on the side to be injected.

Positioning

The patient should be supine, with the head extended and the mouth slightly open to relax the neck muscles. Intravenous access and full monitoring should be instituted.

Dosage

A dose of 10 ml of 0.5 per cent plain bupivacaine, to achieve a prolonged effect (rather than lignocaine).

Equipment

- Resuscitation equipment
- A 21 gauge × 1.5 inch (0.8 × 40 mm) needle, with an extension to allow remote injection
- A 20 ml syringe

Technique

Stellate ganglion block is performed by injection of local anaesthetic into the correct tissue plane. The extent of the block is partly dependent upon the volume injected: small volumes will block the head and neck, while larger volumes will block the arm. There are several approaches to the stellate ganglion, the anterior method being that most commonly used.

1. Palpate between the sternomastoid muscle and the trachea at the level of the cricoid cartilage and identify the C6 transverse process on the side to be injected. Use the index and middle fingers of the other hand to compress the groove between the sternomastoid muscle and the trachea and gently move the carotid sheath laterally; this manoeuvre makes the transverse process more easily palpable.

2. Insert the needle at right angles to the skin to strike the transverse process of C6. If the needle passes too deeply it may enter the vertebral artery or the dural sleeve, or produce tingling in the arm by impinging on the brachial plexus. It is vital that local anaesthetic is not injected unless the operator is sure that the needle is *anterior* to the transverse process. Once the transverse process has been identified, withdraw the needle 2–3 mm, fix the needle, and aspirate to check for the absence of blood or cerebrospinal fluid. Inject a small dose of 0.5 ml of local anaesthetic, and then, if there is no indication of toxicity, slowly inject the total dose.

3. If possible allow the patient to sit up after injection to encourage downward movement of the local anaesthetic. Carefully observe the patient; signs of a correctly placed injection include miosis, enophthalmos, ptosis, suffusion

of the conjunctiva, a blocked nose, a dry, warm skin, and flushing on the side of the injection. However, signs in the head and neck do not confirm that the arm has also been successfully blocked.

Onset and duration

Onset: up to 30 minutes.
Duration: 4–6 hours.

Comments

Stellate ganglion block can produce serious complications and should only be performed by experienced anaesthetists. Injection towards C7 may produce a better block, but it is more hazardous. Bilateral stellate ganglion block should be avoided. Complications include the following

- Haematoma.
- Recurrent laryngeal nerve block occurs in 10 per cent of patients, and produces hoarseness. Because of this, patients should not eat or drink until reflexes return.
- Brachial plexus block and phrenic nerve block can occur.
- Intravascular injection will produce a severe toxic reaction, as the vertebral artery will carry local anaesthetic directly to the brain.
- Aspiration prior to injection cannot guarantee that the needle is not subarachnoid. Injection into a dural sleeve will produce a 'total spinal' anaesthetic, with unconsciousness and cardiopulmonary collapse. Treatment should include oxygenation, intubation and ventilation, a head-down posture, intravenous fluids, and a vasoconstrictor, such as ephedrine.
- Pleural puncture and pneumothorax are potential problems if the needle is either sited too low or directed caudally. If coughing or shortness of breath occur after stellate ganglion block, an expiratory chest film must be taken.
- Osteitis and mediastinitis have been reported, and may occur after oesophageal puncture.

Intercostal block (Fig. 18.3)

Indications

- Analgesia following rib fractures
- Treatment of chest wall pain

Special contraindications

- Intercostal block should not be performed bilaterally
- Obesity
- Contralateral pneumothorax
- Severe airways disease

Anatomy

The intercostal nerves are the anterior primary rami of the thoracic nerves, which leave the intervertebral foramina and

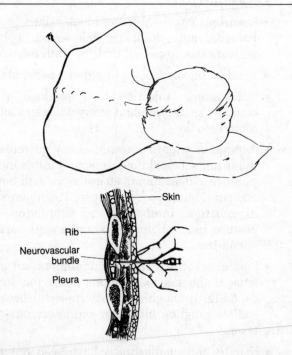

Fig. 18.3 • Intercostal nerve block.

traverse the paravertebral space to run below each rib, together with the intercostal blood vessels. Anteriorly, the neurovascular bundle runs between the external and internal intercostal muscles. The intercostal nerves are sometimes arranged as three or four nerve bundles, rather than a single nerve, and they do not invariably run below the rib margin. Each nerve gives off a lateral branch at the level of the mid-axillary line and an anterior branch near the sternal edge. The upper six intercostal nerves supply the thoracic cage and the lower six nerves also supply the anterior abdominal wall. There is overlap between adjoining segments; consequently, blocking a single intercostal nerve may not produce a segment of altered sensation.

Landmarks

The rib margin must be palpable if the block is to be attempted.

Positioning

The patient lies prone or in the lateral position, with the side to be blocked uppermost. The shoulder should be abducted and the arm should be moved forwards to move the scapula away from the angle of the upper ribs.

Dosage

A dose of 3–5 ml of 1 per cent lignocaine with 1:200 000 adrenaline or 0.375 per cent plain bupivacaine at each level. Intercostal blocks result in high local anaesthetic concentrations in the plasma, because of rapid absorption from the muscle and subpleural space; the toxic dose must not be exceeded.

Equipment

- Resuscitation equipment and a chest drain
- A 23 gauge × 1.25 inch (0.6 × 30 mm) short bevelled needle
- A 5 ml syringe

Technique

The intercostal nerve can be blocked where the rib is palpable at the posterior costal angle at the lateral border of the sacrospinalis muscle, where the intercostal space is at its widest, or just posterior to the mid-axillary line.

1. Instruct the patient to hold his or her breath during needle insertion. Insert the needle perpendicular to the skin, or aim slightly cephalad to strike the lower border of the chosen rib.

2. Withdraw the needle, and redirect it to pass the lower border of the rib to a depth of just 3–4 mm.

3. Aspirate to ensure that air or blood is not present, and inject the local anaesthetic.

Onset and duration

Onset: 5 minutes.
Duration: lignocaine with adrenaline 4–6 hours, bupivacaine 16–20 hours.

Comments

- If the rib is not palpable or cannot be easily contacted with the needle abandon the block, as the risk of pneumothorax is considerable.

- Intercostal block at several levels may be required for multiple rib fractures. Increasing and repeating the number of intercostal blocks performed increases the risk of pneumothorax. It is possible to spread local anaesthetic solution to adjoining segments by injecting a larger volume, for example 20 ml, during a single intercostal block, because the local anaesthetic tracks posteriorly to enter the paravertebral space.

- Patients should be admitted to hospital after intercostal block, as the signs and symptoms of pneumothorax may be delayed for several hours. If the patient coughs or becomes breathless during or after the procedure an expiratory chest radiograph is mandatory.

- Intercostal vessels are commonly punctured during this block, but this does not usually cause problems.

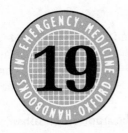

CHAPTER 19

Topical anaesthesia

Topical anaesthesia of the skin

This technique uses EMLA or amethocaine gel.

Indications

- To provide skin anaesthesia, particularly in children.
- Small skin grafts

Special contraindications

- Children less than one year old
- Patients with atopic dermatitis
- Caution should be applied to patients with congenital or acquired methaemoglobinaemia

Dosage

A thick layer of EMLA cream or 4 per cent amethocaine gel should be applied to the area under an occlusive dressing.

Equipment

An occlusive dressing.

Technique

A thick layer of cream is applied to the proposed site(s) of injection. This is covered with an occlusive dressing and left for 1 hour with EMLA or 30 minutes with amethocaine. The procedure should commence within 30 minutes after the dressing has been removed.

Onset and duration

Onset: within 60 minutes (possibly 30 minutes in 1–5 year olds).
Duration: up to 1 hour.

Comments

- EMLA or amethocaine should only be applied to intact skin. It should not be used on wounds or mucous membrane.
- Side-effects include transient local skin blanching or erythema.
- Methaemoglobinaemia in a small child has been reported after EMLA use. In this case 5 g of the cream was applied and left in place for 5 hours.

Ethyl chloride

Ethyl chloride is a clear fluid with a boiling point of 12.5°C. It is stored under pressure in glass containers. It is highly flammable. Local analgesia is obtained by spraying the liquid on to the skin, where it vaporizes, causing a localized area of skin to be cooled rapidly. In the past it was used for minor surgical procedures, such as draining abscesses. It does not provide sufficient analgesia to allow adequate surgical intervention, and should not be used routinely. Occasionally it may be of use when only 'pin-point' analgesia is required. It is best kept locked in a drug cupboard, so that a doctor is likely to think twice before using it.

Topical anaesthesia of the cornea and conjunctiva

Indications

- Removal of a foreign body from the cornea or conjunctiva
- Tonometry

Special contraindications

None.

Anatomy

Corneal sensation is supplied by the short ciliary nerves, with a few fibres from the long ciliary nerves.

Positioning

The patient should sit or lie comfortably, with the head supported.

Dosage

A dose of 1–2 drops for each instillation. Drugs available in single-use packs include 0.5 per cent amethocaine (tetracaine); 1.0 per cent amethocaine (tetracaine); 0.4 per cent oxybuprocaine (benoxinate); 1.0 per cent lignocaine and fluorescein 0.25 per cent; 0.5 per cent proxymetacaine.

Technique

Instillation may be performed in two ways.

1. With the patient looking down, raise the upper eyelid and instil two drops on to the eye.
2. With the patient looking up, pull the lower eyelid down and instil two drops on to the eye.

The initial instillation is often accompanied by a stinging sensation, which wears off after about 30 seconds. At this time a further two drops should be instilled into the eye.

Onset and duration

Onset: within 30 seconds.
Duration: variable. Proxymetacaine will persist for an average of 15 minutes.

Comments

- Always check if the patient is allergic to a particular local anaesthetic. This may be due to the local anaesthetic itself or to a preservative. Hypersensitivity commonly presents as conjunctivitis and dermatitis.

- Always protect the anaesthetized eye from trauma and foreign bodies for a minimum of 6 hours. This is usually done using a double eye pad. Remember that if local anaesthetic is put in both eyes at the same time both will need protection. Goggles may be used, so that the patient can still see.

- Amethocaine is hydrolysed in the body to *p*-aminobenzoic acid and should therefore not be used in patients being treated with sulphonamides.

- Proxymetacaine causes less stinging and may be useful in children.

- In obtaining a satisfactory level of anaesthesia, the number of instillations is of far greater importance than the amount of local anaesthetic used for each instillation.

Topical anaesthesia of the larynx and trachea

Indications

To allow tracheal intubation or bronchoscopy in patients in whom general anaesthesia is not possible. It may be used as a way of securing the airway, yet avoiding the use of muscle-relaxants. Carefully chosen patients with chest disease, skeletal or neuromuscular disorders, or trauma may benefit from awake intubation under local anaesthesia.

Special contraindications

- Local anaesthesia does not obtund the cardiovascular response to intubation and it is therefore not appropriate in patients with myocardial ischaemia, hypertension, cerebrovascular disease, or raised intracranial pressure.

- Local anaesthetics in the airway depress the cough reflex and must never be given to patients where there is a risk of blood, pus, or gastric contents entering the pharynx. It must not be used in the unfasted patient.

Anatomy

The superior and recurrent laryngeal branches of the vagus nerves provide the sensory supply to the larynx, trachea, and bronchi. The superior laryngeal nerve passes deep to the carotid artery and divides into a small external branch and a large internal branch; the latter pierces the thyrohyoid membrane above the superior laryngeal artery to supply the laryngeal surface of the epiglottis, the aryepiglottic folds, and the interior of the larynx as far down as the vocal cords. The inferior branch of the recurrent laryngeal nerve approaches the larynx in the groove between the oesophagus and the trachea, with the laryngeal branch of the inferior thyroid artery to supply the mucosa of the larynx below the cords, the trachea, and the bronchi.

Landmarks

The cricothyroid membrane is palpated in the midline to perform transtracheal injection.

Positioning

The patient lies in a supine position, with the head resting on one pillow.

Dosage

A total of 5 ml of 4 per cent lignocaine (40 mg/ml) or 20 sprays of 10 per cent lignocaine aerosol (10 mg/spray) may be used. Combinations of the two preparations can be used, but the total dose must be carefully calculated, as local anaesthetics are readily absorbed from mucous membranes.

Equipment

- A 10 per cent lignocaine aerosol or 4 per cent lignocaine in a suitable spray
- Two small swabs soaked in 4 per cent lignocaine
- Curved forceps
- A 2 ml syringe containing 4 per cent lignocaine with a 23 gauge 1.25 inch (0.6 × 30 mm) needle, a laryngoscope, and tracheal tubes

Technique

1. Spray the mouth and pharynx with a small amount of 4 per cent or 10 per cent lignocaine and wait 2–3 minutes.

2. Gently introduce the laryngoscope over the tongue and spray a further dose of lignocaine more posteriorly.

3. Anaesthetize the internal branches of the superior laryngeal nerves, where they pass beneath the mucosa of the pyriform fossae, by passing a local anaesthetic-soaked swab, held in curved forceps, over the back of the tongue, holding it in position for 2 minutes on each side. A superior hyoid injection can be used as an alternative.

4. View the glottis using a laryngoscope. Spray 4 per cent lignocaine on to the glottis and allow it to run into the trachea.

5. If laryngoscopy is not possible use transtracheal injection to anaesthetize the trachea. Extend the patient's head and advance a 23 gauge needle through the cricothyroid membrane, perpendicularly and in the midline, until air is aspirated, confirming that the needle-tip is in the trachea. Inject 2 ml of 4 per cent lignocaine at the end of expiration and quickly withdraw the needle. (Lignocaine entering the trachea causes the patient to cough, which disperses the local anaesthetic.)

Onset and duration

Onset: 2–5 minutes.
Duration: 2–3 hours.

Comments

- Patients must not eat or drink for 3 hours after local anaesthesia to the larynx, because of the risk of aspiration.

- While awake intubation under local anaesthesia is a valuable technique, it requires practice and is potentially hazardous; it should only be performed by experienced anaesthetists.

- Possible complications include needle breakage, subcutaneous emphysema, vocal cord damage, and inadvertent submucosal injection leading to airway obstruction.

Cricothyroid puncture is contraindicated in the presence of bleeding disorders, local sepsis, or tumour.

Topical anaesthesia of the urethra

Indications

Catheterization.

Special contraindications

Bulbo-cavernous reflux.

Anatomy

The urethra is supplied by branches of the perineal nerve.

Positioning

The patient lies supine.

Dosage

Men: 15 ml lignocaine gel.
Women: 3–5 ml lignocaine gel.
(1 ml lignocaine gel contains 21.4 mg lignocaine hydrochloride.)

Equipment

A prepacked tube of local anaesthetic gel with nozzle or an accordion syringe with local anaesthetic gel.

Technique

Male

The penile part of the urethra is filled first, by instilling 10 ml of the local anaesthetic into the urethra. Ask the patient to strain, as if passing urine, and inject a further 5 ml to fill the posterior urethra.

Female

Inject 3 to 5 ml of local anaesthetic into the urethra.

Onset and duration

Onset: 4–5 minutes.
Duration: 2–3 hours.

Comments

- Aqueous local anaesthetic preparations may be used. The gel preparations have the advantage of providing lubrication for instrumentation. They also remain in contact longer with the mucous membrane and so may prolong the duration of action.
- Local anaesthetic toxicity may occur if there is mucosal damage. Care must be taken if there is bleeding from the meatus. A few patients may have a bulbo-cavernous connection, and instillation under high pressure may cause injection directly into the blood stream.
- Some aqueous and gel preparations contain preservatives to which patients may be allergic. Antiseptic agents may also be added to the gels.

Index